PRAISE FOR *MUSE*

Hear from women, in their own words, who have both read *Muse* and worked with Dr. Amanda Hanson on the power of reclaiming our womanhood.

"The invaluable teachings of Dr. Amanda Hanson will unlock the doors you have been trapped behind. The wisdom in this book will remind you that you have held the keys all along, how to use these keys, how to find them when they slip from your hands in the dark moments, and how to step out of the cage entirely as your truest, most authentic self."

—DIANNA HAMPTON

"The word *life-changing* is often overused and exaggerated and so I am reticent and careful in using this word. But there is simply no other way to describe working with Dr Amanda Hanson. She has equipped me with the tools and knowledge that have both grown my inner strength and gently pushed me to challenge the ideals imparted on me by society and to uncover my own truth. She cares so very deeply about her clients and creates the most beautiful of safe spaces, free of judgement, where you can explore who you really are and work deeply on yourself and your relationship with others. I feel very fortunate to be working with someone whom I admire and who gives a voice, and a platform, to women."

—MARCIA GENJELIAN

"Working with Amanda and infusing her beautiful practices into my daily routine has given me a jump start on life. Not only has it allowed me to heal the wounded areas in myself, but I can now also proactively combat any message that otherwise tells me I should not love who I am or live to my fullest expression. With all of this, I have the self-confidence and self-trust necessary to exist as my most beautiful, authentic, rich and confident self—a version of myself I never thought I would be able to attain. Read this book and become who you were meant to be."

—EMMA DAVIS

"Dr. Amanda Hanson will empower you to chart the map back to yourself, the 'you' you had forgotten. She will invite and seduce you to realign with your divine power, transcend trauma, and trespass on what has been before today. She will rekindle the fire inside you that you had forgotten to tend to."

—ANDREEA MILLER

"In June of 2024 my life shifted after meeting Dr. Amanda Hanson. I am the voice of a fifty-nine-year-old woman who was completely unaware how the patriarchy ruled my existence, keeping me separated from the magnificent female goddess I was put on this earth to be. As I walk this journey of the divine feminine, I am learning to embrace grief, rage, sensuality, joy, and love of myself. Is it easy? Absolutely not. Is it life changing? It absolutely is. Dr. Amanda Hanson says, 'Even if you can only give 1 percent a day, you are making a change.' Some days I can only give 1 percent to myself but most days I give a lot more. Please join us on the journey of female self-empowerment so that we can share this message and help all the sisters of the world rise."

—CAROL ZOLLER

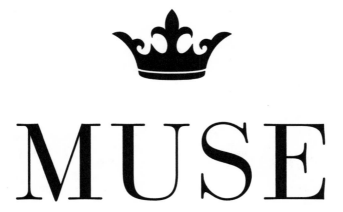

MUSE

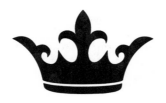

MUSE

THE MAGNETISM OF WOMEN WHO STOP ABANDONING THEMSELVES

DR. AMANDA HANSON

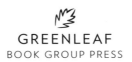

GREENLEAF
BOOK GROUP PRESS

This book is not meant to diagnose or treat any medical or psychological conditions and is not a substitute for seeking professional help and treatment. Readers using the information in this book do so entirely at their own risk, and the author and publisher accept no liability if adverse effects are caused.

Published by Greenleaf Book Group Press
Austin, Texas
www.gbgpress.com

Distributed by Greenleaf Book Group

For ordering information or special discounts for bulk purchases, please contact Greenleaf Book Group at PO Box 91869, Austin, TX 78709, 512.891.6100.

Design and composition by Greenleaf Book Group and Sheila Parr
Cover design by Greenleaf Book Group and Sheila Parr

Publisher's Cataloging-in-Publication data is available.

Print ISBN: 979-8-88645-318-8

eBook ISBN: 979-8-88645-319-5

To offset the number of trees consumed in the printing of our books, Greenleaf donates a portion of the proceeds from each printing to the Arbor Day Foundation. Greenleaf Book Group has replaced over 50,000 trees since 2007.

Printed in the United States of America on acid-free paper
25 26 27 28 29 30 31 32   10 9 8 7 6 5 4 3 2 1
First Edition

To all women who know there is a more beautiful way—
most especially Ava, who has already begun.

CONTENTS

Introduction

YOUR INVITATION TO REDEFINE WOMANHOOD

MY DEAR MUSE,

I invite you to think of the last time you looked at yourself in the mirror. Maybe as you got ready for the day, applying makeup and doing your hair. Or as you caught sight of yourself in a hallway mirror at home or in the office. Or as you got ready for bed, after washing your face or while brushing your teeth.

Tell me: As you studied the reflection before you, what did you see, think, and feel?

I hope you met yourself straight in the eyes and felt deep love for the woman looking back at you. I hope you embraced the wisdom each line represents, celebrated the architecture of your natural skin, and felt wonder at your exceptional hair and changing facial shape. I hope you smiled at yourself and said out loud: "I love you. You are beautiful and perfect."

My greatest desire is that you met yourself in the mirror and felt reverence. And if so, I celebrate you, because as a woman in this modern world, you've arrived at a remarkable space—self-acceptance—which most women never reach. After reading this book, you will understand why.

More commonly, women avoid their own gaze. As they look into the mirror, they pull at their skin and touch their hair in disgust, using makeup and potions to shape-shift into society's definition of a beautiful, supple woman. Worse yet, most women leave this encounter with their reflection feeling worthless.

Imperfect.

Ugly.

Aging.

Even invisible.

And if this is truer to your experience, I celebrate you, too, because you made the most healing and radical act by picking up this book. You've taken the first step on a journey toward connecting with the sacred, worthy, and radiant woman not just in the mirror, but more importantly: within you.

I know, because I've witnessed hundreds of women taking this journey throughout the more than twenty-five years I've spent dedicated to my work as a clinical psychologist. During that time, I've worked with women across the globe, as well as impacted millions with content I've created around celebrating aging, rejecting patriarchy, learning to trust their intuition, digging deep to understand their true desires, and building an unshakable foundation of self-worth.

I've heard endless stories of women who ache for more emotional intimacy with their partners, who want collaborative decision-making in the household, who desire to experience lovemaking with eye contact, and who crave weekends without alcohol. Women who speak of wanting to worry less about how they look and more about how they feel. Who long for friendships in which conversations don't begin with, "You look like you lost weight," but instead with, "How is your heart?"

When they begin working with me and we have these conversations about beliefs and meaning, the "off" feeling begins to make sense. I watch women start to put the pieces of the puzzle together, the years of confusion clicking into place with clarity. The light returns to their eyes.

I want that for you, too.

While the symptoms of each of my clients were entirely different, all of these women had something in common. Despite their religion, origin, upbringing, financial situation, marital status, traumas, or anything else, all—and I mean *all*—of these women were at war with themselves.

When I asked them the question I asked you, about their last encounter with themselves in the mirror, each reported looking at their bodies through a critical lens. As we dug deeper, it became clear that this constant self-criticism had nothing to do with their actual physical shape, condition, or age, because they all admitted that this critique had been there as long as they can remember. All of these women struggled with their sense of self-worth, as though they contained an unseen filter that hid their humanity from themselves, leaving them with ever-present self-loathing over physical qualities that didn't fit the ideal they saw on all the screens around them.

In my exploration of these women's journeys, I also found that every single one of them experienced a similar event roughly around the age of nine years old—some women as early as six or as late as twelve—that forever shaped their perception of what "ideal" means to them. That event? Typically, it was a comment from a close relative or friend about their body. A comment that, for the first time in their young lives, made them see themselves through a critical lens. A comment that shifted, forever, how they saw themselves.

This is true for my clients, and in the conversations I've had with women across the globe, I've found that most women clearly remember this moment and the specific comment that changed their self-view. Some can even repeat it word for word. It pierces them so deeply that, no matter how much positive feedback or compliments they receive later in life, the verbal wound remains. It scars but does not heal.

This early memory is a formative, shared experience for nearly all of us women. It is one of our earliest lessons about self-worth. The experience signals that, from now on, the way we feel about ourselves depends on the perception of the outside world. That initial critique becomes the guide for how we measure our worthiness. It becomes an integrated inner voice that then speaks with us as we are standing in front of the mirror.

We turn twenty, thirty, forty, fifty years old and beyond . . . and we never examine that voice. We never even stop to question why it's there.

THIS JOURNEY CAN BE SCARY

By the end of this book, you will have a clear understanding of your inner voice. You'll know how those early experiences are a part of a bigger scheme designed to stifle your self-worth. You'll begin noticing how the environment around you is designed to make you believe your body is not good enough. That you are not smart enough or worthy enough.

And most importantly, by the end of this book, you will possess all the necessary tools to exit that race, and to meet yourself with honor, reverence, and power.

Everything I share in this book is based on facts, data, my personal experience, and the experiences of hundreds of women that I've worked with. But first, a warning label: This book might make you more radical. It might trigger you and make you feel overwhelmed. And importantly, this book will cause you to look at yourself through a completely different lens, and therefore make informed decisions about your body, spirit, and mind. You can't unlearn what you're about to know.

I understand this journey of awareness and change, not just in working with my clients over the past two-plus decades but also from personal experience. I have personally walked the path before you. This book details my own journey of opting out of posing for the system and into claiming unapologetic self-worth rooted to my own decision-making. I will take you to the most vulnerable parts of my life and share the most intense transformations that enabled me to become immune to the traps of patriarchy and toxic beauty culture later in life, as I aged into my silver hair and wise wrinkles.

But while I write this as an anchored woman today, I promise to be honest with you about the parts of my experience that have been hard. Because this journey has been scary, in so many ways.

Opting out of what the majority of people never even question is scary. Finding your own way, with no one leading you with certainty, is scary. Not always having the end goal in mind is scary.

But as I'm writing this book at the age of fifty-one, I'm standing together with millions of women who resonated with my message when I first began publicly speaking about aging, self-worth, and the sacredness of being a woman. These messages have resonated with women of all walks of life, in every corner of our globe.

I hope this book resonates with you in much the same way. Many parts of this book will feel like remembering an ancient wisdom that lives within you. Trust those feelings.

The best news: unlike me, you are not going this alone. When you say yes to this journey, you step into an incredible sisterhood that wants to see you strive in your truth, authenticity, and health. And while this journey continues long after you finish this book, please know you are now connected to the thousands of women who know exactly how you feel, desire what you crave, and have that same inner knowing of deserving more.

You are not alone. You are with your sisters, including me. Let's begin.

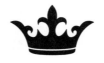

Section I

CREATING CONTEXT
FOR THE SUFFERING

Chapter 1

CONSCIOUS MATRIARCHY

"Women grow more radical with age."
—GLORIA STEINEM

"ARE YOU GETTING Botox anytime soon?" My friend studied me across the restaurant table, waiting for a reply to what she seemed to think was the most normal question in the world.

But it was not a normal question to me. Botox? I was forty years old, having just celebrated entering a new decade only a few months prior. Was she seriously asking if I was going to inject a foreign substance—a poison—into my face to look younger?

My friend continued to watch me, shifting in her chair at the uncomfortable silence.

"Getting what?" was all I could find as a response.

The rest of our conversation that day felt stilted. Unbalanced. She shared how she didn't even want to celebrate her upcoming birthday. The forties weren't worth celebrating, she explained. She bemoaned her age and her body and looked at me every time she degraded herself, as if expecting me to do the same. I'm sure I looked like a blank-brained doll looking back at her, confused, thinking about my own face and body and how I liked them just fine.

But should I? Was there something wrong with the most natural process in the world—aging? Suddenly, I felt not just disconnected from my friend but also disconnected from myself.

That day, something shifted inside me. It was as if someone spun my head around to confront a part of a reality I had never seen, or at least had never paid attention to.

And I know I'm not alone. During my twenty-five years as a clinical psychologist, not to mention the thousands of personal conversations I've had by now as a woman of fifty-one, I know that every woman experiences a moment—perhaps many—like mine that afternoon at the restaurant. The question may be posed by a friend or a reel on social media or a flippant comment in an episode on television. It might be suggested by a dermatologist or in an ad online. At some point, every woman is confronted with the question: Will you do everything in your power to freeze time, to preserve your youth?

Act now! society insists. Once your beauty is gone, it's gone!

We get this messaging from the time we are very young, even before we have grown into pimples. Women are bombarded with messages of worth being tied to beauty from as early as we can understand language. We'll unpack that later. For now, I want to focus on my conversation at that table and what happened after, a representative experience that takes different shapes for different women but happens everywhere, all around the world.

I said goodbye to my friend that day, hugging her like normal but walking away feeling doom settling into my abdomen, like a festering sickness I needed to purge. And from that day on, the number of conversations about antiaging procedures multiplied. I watched women around me tug at their chins and midsections and bemoan their changing bodies, and within a short time, conversations with my friends changed completely. We didn't speak about our dreams and who we aspired to become anymore, even when I tried to edge conversations toward those topics. More often, women discussed how frequently they were coloring their gray, how they were staying out of the sun from now on, and how they were sleeping on their backs to avoid getting chest wrinkles. One girlfriend even requested a facelift from her husband for her fiftieth birthday!

I felt like I was getting zapped by fear from every angle, popped straight out of my safe bubble and forced to confront the fear of aging around me. I was confused at the absurdity of it all. Just the year before, we were having conversations about our biggest plans; now, we are picking at our bodies.

What was happening? Why wasn't I worried about my wrinkles, my shifting body, my age? Was I missing something?

At the heart of my questioning was a creeping fear, something I hadn't thought of until these conversations began: Does visibly aging decrease a woman's value? Should I fear aging?

DOES MIDLIFE HAVE TO BE ALL NEGATIVE?

I'd never questioned my value as a woman before, at least not to this extent. But suddenly, I was questioning everything. While I inherently rejected a fear of aging, I also knew I needed to understand these fears to combat them—for myself, my clients, and my own daughter. I needed to form my own philosophy, to discover my own definition of aging so I could confidently move into these next decades of life feeling anchored and whole, and help the women around me do the same. Or at least the ones who were willing to have these conversations.

So I got curious. And as one does with such curiosities, I turned to Google.

One afternoon not long after that life-shifting conversation with my friend, I sat down at my computer to learn more about midlife. I was hoping to find a collective or a powerful female leader—something, *anything* hopeful that would counter the fear about this time in our lives. I wanted to find a new narrative, one that inspired me and that I could share with others.

Yet as I typed the word "midlife" into the search bar, I drew in a quick breath as I stared in dismay at the auto-filled word "crisis." Dejected, I hit the return bar on my keyboard and scrolled through the results before me, becoming increasingly deflated and insulted.

Article after article detailed the perils of aging—decline in memory, focus, and the ability to learn new things.[1] Menopausal women can experience issues with incontinence, pain during intercourse, and insomnia, with negative effects lasting for years.

And alongside the many, many articles about the perils of midlife for women, I found endless products, skin care routines, and procedures promising to maintain a "youthful" appearance. Hormone treatments, injections, creams . . . the options were endless.

Where were the stories of the incredible transformations and experiences that come with aging? Why could I not find one single article about the beauty of aging and what this time can represent in a woman's life? Why was there nothing that teaches us to focus on our souls, and on navigating this momentous life stage with presence and self-love? Where were the studies and wisdom I could share with the women who came to my psychology practice in search of more meaning, depth, and reimagining their next chapter?

Instead, the message was clear: Make sure no one can see that you're aging. Freeze your external body. Inject and manipulate; starve and medicate. No one wants to see your wrinkles. No one wants to look at an aging woman.

I was hoping to find midlife magic; instead, I found a singular message: Aging as a woman is a crisis. I sat back from my computer and pushed the keyboard away in disgust.

Is this as good as it gets? I wondered. A decade of hot flashes, sagging skin, dry vagina, confusion, unhappiness, antiaging quick-fixes, and our best years in the rearview mirror, with nothing to look forward to?

Slowly I felt my inner light start to dim. That sparkle that had carried me through the poverty of my youth and through my doctorate in psychology, the confidence I'd held about my worth as a woman being based on my character and actions, the intense love I felt for life . . . I could feel it slipping.

But I couldn't let that happen. I needed to figure out a way to combat what I saw as a festering infection of fear.

While I wasn't looking to bypass the physical realities of menopause, I knew it was critical for me to have something to look forward to. Without another narrative of aging—a more balanced philosophy—midlife would feel like I was gripping my seat, waiting for hell to begin.

So my wondering shifted: Could aging as a woman feel anchored? Spiritual? Even holy?

> *Is this as good as it gets? A decade of hot flashes, sagging skin, dry vagina, confusion, unhappiness, antiaging quick-fixes, and our best years in the rearview mirror, with nothing to look forward to?*

REJECT FEAR, RECLAIM YOUR LIFE, REWRITE YOUR BELIEFS

Sitting there at my desk, these thoughts swirling, my mind trying to make sense of what I'd found, I didn't know yet how this moment would change my life. That I was about to uncover an entire system designed to keep women depleted. That my burgeoning philosophy—the spirituality of aging—would go on to help women across the globe. Or that sharing this knowledge online would spark a movement of millions of women joining hands with me to reject the fear of aging and reclaim their lives.

From that moment, this book was born. It would, of course, take many years for my message to take hold and for all of these things to happen.

I wrote this book to bring back the honor of being a woman. To help foster critical thinking. To offer a new path toward aging—one that is spiritual. Beautiful. Anchored. Calm. Self-loving. If you stick with me throughout this book, that's my promise: You'll learn to love yourself.

Up until now, I bet no one in your life has sat you down for a real, hard conversation about aging. The discussions you've had up until now have likely been like mine were, about keeping the visibility of our aging bodies at bay—whispers about procedures and skincare routines and exercises to stave off belly-fat.

Or maybe you're on the other side of the conversation, with women who have decided to give up, to not try anymore, who have decided they're too old or too fat or too ugly or too worthless. You're hearing sentences that start with phrases like "at my age" and end with self-degradation. Worst of all, they expect you to join them.

Or maybe you're not quite into these conversations yet, still in what society defines as the peak of life, the supple beauty of youth, yet you still don't love yourself and you're terrified of losing your value as you age. You have no strong female example around you, not a single one, who loves herself. And you know that you want a more beautiful future, one where you look in the mirror and see your biggest support and best friend looking back at you, a woman who truly adores you.

This book will bring you on a journey of letting go of the fear of aging and leaning into self-love. Throughout the pages of this book, we will detail the history of why we are here and how we can journey into a new, revolutionary womanhood. You'll learn to anchor into self-trust. You'll reconnect to your inner knowing and begin making anchored decisions from a place of self-awareness.

You'll rewrite your beliefs. You'll create self-honor. You'll learn about your holy body—its cycles and seasons—from both a biological and spiritual sense, and how to honor your needs. You'll cultivate sensuality and self-intimacy. You'll exit the endless gratitude trap and learn how to welcome in desire for more.

But first: a warning label. This book will trigger you. I will share stories that will make you deeply uncomfortable. There might be moments where you want nothing more to do with this book—maybe even throw it across the room in disgust.

That's OK. I decided long ago that my work in the world would be honest. But I want you to know that every single thing I share in this book comes from a place of love for you. A place that wants you to experience the most beautiful, full, loving life possible. And if you journey with me, if you stick through those hardest parts, if you try even a sliver of the activities in this book, if you approach this work with openness, I promise you'll arrive on the other side as a different woman. Because what we're about to explore can't be unseen. The known can't be unknown.

That's my promise to you: to be real, to challenge you, to give you not only facts and data but also lived experiences from real women, including myself. To provide the examples I didn't have but desperately needed. To guide you toward a sisterhood, a movement: the spirituality of aging.

FINDING YOUR SISTERHOOD

This book began as a battle cry for women in midlife. But while writing the book, I changed course as I heard from thousands of women in their twenties and thirties already facing the inherent pressures of remaining forever youthful—even in their youth.

My urgency to shift and expand this book grew as I deeply understood that women today start the internal war and punishment even sooner than previous generations. Botox as a twenty-first birthday gift from mom. Labiaplasty to change the look of the vulva for girls under twenty-five. College girls afraid of sun damage and lip wrinkles from using straws. Even well before a woman visibly ages, society has done such a remarkable job promoting dread that she approaches aging with a sense of fear and lack.

Living with this negative energy swirling in one's psyche impacts everything: relationships, feelings of worthiness, and self-respect. One cannot fully experience the beauty of life while constantly searching for validation. Functioning from a place of scarcity steals the ability to wholly live in the present moment and to connect with each other. Part of the antidote to this disconnect is having an aligned sisterhood—a group of women with whom you can share the richness of life. Finding this support made all the difference for me.

HOW I FOUND MY SISTERHOOD

As I mentioned earlier, in my early forties, when I found myself surrounded by incredible women who were completely preoccupied with fear—including my friend who asked me about Botox—I knew I needed more. Our time together was wasted on complaints about their wrinkles, what med spa was the best in town, and what antiaging serum seemed most effective. I was bored, disheartened, and craved more from my relationships. I wanted to know who they desired to become in their second act. What they were dreaming about. What made their hearts race. How they would write this chapter of life. But all of my attempts to switch the conversation were met with confusion and disregard.

As time went on, my loneliness grew. I could be in a group of women yet feel completely alone and disconnected. For the first time, I felt like my friends and I were speaking two different languages. I was unwilling to be consumed by the fear of aging, and they were convinced that from this point on their value was declining, unless they figured out how to maintain a youthful appearance. Over time, my sadness morphed into frustration and anger. I was losing my girlfriends—smart, funny, big-hearted, incredible women—to the fears of aging. And as much as I had loved our years together, I knew I couldn't swim in that toxic water or it would poison me too. I had to find another pond to swim in.

I reasoned that there must be other women who were committed to making midlife the most magnificent, epic stage of their lives. Women who craved deeper conversations. Women who cared about their evolving souls more than their changing bodies—and who revered those changes. Women who wanted to talk about world issues, matters of the heart, and the future of humanity.

I ached for like-minded women to share life with.

One day, as I was driving home from a women's retreat, I knew I could no longer keep up the charade. I needed more. In that moment, I declared to myself that I would find women who wanted to have bigger conversations— women who craved more soulful adventures and who could celebrate aging.

The next day, I posted a brief video in a Facebook group of local moms, saying I was interested in meeting women who wanted to gather and share deeper conversations and connections. I said I'd be opening my home the following Thursday evening and invited anyone interested to message me. To my elation, 120 women responded and 67 showed up. I asked those who arrived with the customary host gift of wine to leave it near the front door and grab it on their way out, because I had made a conscious decision to keep this evening alcohol-free. I wanted to have meaningful conversations that included authentic vulnerability, not the falsified truth-telling alcohol enables. When the next gathering was more intimate, with 32 women, I wondered if some women were uncomfortable without wine culture as a barrier remover.

Think about this: How often in our lives do we speak about our most vulnerable matters without a sip of alcohol?

I can't adequately put into words how incredible those evenings were in the presence of so many women. While I could have never imagined where these initial gatherings would lead me, I knew that every cell in my body was fully activated, and I wanted to feel this way forever.

I didn't feel lonely anymore. I felt like I had found a sisterhood.

We continued to gather for six more months, with each meetup having a specific theme. Every month, I would spend hours transforming my family room and kitchen into a sacred space for community. I carried every book I owned into the kitchen and placed them on my dinner table for the women to peruse. I made beautiful fruit and vegetable platters and lined my counter with crackers, chocolates, and bottled water. I put out my favorite leather box and a stack of blank pieces of paper and pens next to it, with a note leaning against the box that said: "Let me know about future topics you would like us to discuss. You can remain anonymous."

It was fascinating and revealing to learn what the women hungered to talk about: dying parents, sex in long-term relationships, divorce, identity, racism, LGBTQ+ issues, gun violence, solo traveling, literature. Not once did I see a request to talk about Botox.

Our conversations were deep. We discussed how women can claim their voices. We debated the art of communicating so your needs are heard and respected. We talked about relationships with our mothers and how to break the legacy of suffering. We explored how to choose love over fear in humanity, especially when it comes to issues of diversity. I even brought in an occasional speaker to add variety to the format.

After each meetup, women left notes of thanks, reflecting on how desperately they had been longing for such gatherings and how fulfilling it was for them to connect with other women. Soon, I became more than just fulfilled; I realized I had found the calling for my life's second act. While I'd been working one-on-one with clients for decades as a psychologist, the energy of guiding a powerful group of women lit something new within me. I knew I would spend the rest of my life gathering women together to talk about the matters of our hearts. I felt an inner tug to expand beyond my living room, to help even more women feel such an awakening.

Looking around the room each month, I witnessed women at all stages of life who were leaning into the experience of womanhood. They were opening up with vulnerability and inviting connection, with themselves and with others. And for each time, each month, each topic, each woman I greeted at my front door—well, I nearly burst wide open with gratitude. I had been so low, tiptoeing toward fear of aging. What a relief to have pushed away those fears—dominated by patriarchy and objectification—and to have instead stepped into the next phase of my life with power and presence.

And to surround myself with women who did the same!

This experience, and many experiences after, taught me an important lesson: Your sisterhood exists, no matter what you are going through.

It's just that sometimes you have to become the leader who calls other women in. You can attract women who celebrate and dream with you, who see aging as a spiritual journey and approach it with deep reverence. It starts internally, with the journey you're about to take in this book; it continues by shedding the fear of connecting with other women, the fear of rejection, and deciding to bond through vulnerable conversations about topics that really matter to you. Because when you show up in the vibrancy of your worth, these women will come. When you show up in self-love, you'll attract women who are self-loving.

You don't need to host dozens of women in your home. Leadership can start with yourself. It begins with seeing your body and soul through a lens of love. Because self-love will ensure the rejection of fear, and rejection of fear will attract women who are celebrating life, who enjoy their days, and who love the experience of being a woman. And aren't those the most incredible shared values that a friendship can be based on?

Now tell me: In such a community, with such girlfriends, is aging a crisis? Or is it magic?

REJECTING TOXIC "BEAUTY CULTURE"

Along with community, the road to rooted womanhood requires rejecting much of the world's messaging. After all, we live in a culture that sells a toxic promise: eternal youthfulness. Or as it's referred to by most people, beauty culture.

While many women believe females define and own female beauty, the truth is we live in a world that was created by men for men. While there is some nuance to this statement, the more you dig into modern society—what we buy, watch, wear, do with our time, and engage in nearly every aspect of our female experience—the fact is, nearly all of it is created with men in mind.

To set the stage for our journey in this book, we must first explore beauty.

What is beauty? Have you ever stopped to consider this concept, and what it holds for you in your life? Or is it something you measure yourself by in the mirror each day, via unrealistic expectations set by society and internalized within yourself?

From a purely definitional sense, beauty pleases the senses. It catches our attention and causes us to feel a rush of pleasure and appreciation. Beauty has been a driving force for centuries—we see records and measures of beauty in our earliest art. While we often consider beauty to be objective, the truth is beauty standards change. As quoted in a 1987 article in the *Washington Post*, "Faces go in and out of fashion."[2] And the beauty in favor reflects the power structures in society.

It was true when that article was published in the 1980s and it was true in ancient times as well. Classical Roman and Greek statues, for example, feature lines inspired by realistic male and female bodies. Consider the classic sculpture *Venus de' Medici*. You've probably seen images of this marble rendition of the goddess Venus: a life-size female, nude, with a hand partially covering one breast and a hand covering her genitals. Created around the first century BCE, her age is ambiguous—she could be twenty or fifty. The statue has a belly and wide hips. Its features are soft, not angular or sharp: jaw, arms, midsection, legs. This body type was esteemed as the epitome of beauty among depictions of the goddess of love and beauty.

Now, fast-forward to the 1960s and '70s, when there was a notable shift in beauty standards for women, transitioning from the mature, voluptuous physique represented by icons like Marilyn Monroe to the slender, flat-chested silhouette popularized by supermodels such as Twiggy. What's most striking is that as women made significant strides in education, employment, and politics, the ideal female body began to take up less space.

Moving further forward to the modern day, one 2019 survey of one thousand Americans revealed that the "perfect" woman is described as five feet, five inches tall and 128 pounds, with a twenty-six-inch waist.[3] Yet according to data collected by the US CDC—Centers for Disease Control and Prevention—the average female adult is only five feet, three-and-a-half inches tall and weighs about 170 pounds, with a nearly thirty-nine-inch waist. Talk about unrealistic idealization![4]

Those unattainable standards apply to youthfulness too. Scientific researchers have studied the double standard of aging, that is, men's perceived value grows but women's declines as they age. One study in the *Journal of Aging Studies* reveals that the impact is even more pronounced by class, with lower socioeconomic status being associated with less confidence in aging and higher socioeconomic status facing added pressure related to appearance.[5] Neither of those situations sound desirable to me.

These feelings are compounded by the products advertised by celebrities, influencers, and thought leaders. Just look at their perfect skin with no sign of aging or imperfections on their faces! We know, intellectually, that they are assisted by procedures, makeup, and camera filters, not to mention the magic of Photoshop. But I'll bet that logic doesn't prevent you from making comparisons or feeling a pang of unworthiness when you see these "perfect" images.

When a beauty standard becomes self-terrorizing, health-threatening, unattainable, and dismantling, it is no longer a standard of beauty—it's what I call a toxic beauty standard.

The trouble is these standards are pervasive. They're everywhere, in every magazine, on every website, in every social media feed. And the more exposure you have to them, the sooner they spread. They're like a virus that grips your system and won't let go. But this virus doesn't cause stomach aches or fever; it causes a drop in self-esteem. And from this place of lack, women desperately search for approval. This is why the average woman's self-esteem is close to non-existent. The worst part? Physical youthfulness gets further away every day, which means the effort increases every day, week, month, year, decade.

Aside from the emotional toll, the danger of superficial youthfulness is that, after a certain age, "preventing" aging has nothing to do with health. Women undergo dangerous procedures, inject toxins into their faces, stuff their bodies into organ-restrictive garments, take dangerous weight loss medications, and risk their lives just to stay relevant. What do you think a woman's life journey will feel like if she believes her value is declining with every year? The obvious answer: not great. Fraught with inner pain. Lacking in self-love.

With the global beauty market set to reach $580 billion by 2027, companies are motivated to keep us believing this storyline.[6] After all, toxic beauty culture must manufacture fear to sell its goods, because its sole purpose is to market a solution to a made-up problem. Consequently, corporations must create a story of lack and terror around getting older, or they won't be able to sell their products and make those billions of dollars.

Advertisers need us to be ashamed of our sizes, faces, odors, hair, voices, nails, age, feelings, and desires. It seems the only thing we *shouldn't* be ashamed of is lack of self-esteem. Because that place of lack leads to spending: seeking more unhealthy transformations that could cause irreversible damage.

God forbid you question the system or decide to opt out. The shame.

And we women are participating. When we spend our money on changing our bodies to fit toxic beauty standards, we participate in the system.

When we resign ourselves to injections and starvation and hundreds of dollars in lotions and potions, we support toxic beauty culture. When we comment on other women's faces and bodies, or even our own sacred selves, we participate in it as well. We vote for these standards with our money and our words. And breaking that cycle requires us to vote differently.

I experienced what this change in party lines can look like recently during a trip to Positano, Italy. During my three weeks in the Italian village, I witnessed European women taking great pride in their appearance with their silver hair, beautiful lines, and exquisite character etched across every part of their faces. They often expressed themselves through clothing, makeup, and hair. The women I met didn't seem to wear their makeup as a mask—rather, they seemed to take pride in enhancing their natural beauty. And they were stunning.

This is what I want for you: to let go of the storyline given in the United States and perpetuated globally, and opt into the natural beauty that already exists within you. To reconnect with the younger you, the child who learned that the most valuable thing you have to offer is your beauty. I want you to stop spending your precious life contorting, starving, silencing, and complying—just so that you feel loved, chosen, and approved of by everyone other than yourself. I want you to stop trading your big dreams for conformity.

And mostly: I pray this book is your reclamation. That reading these pages represents your decision to take back the truth. That by opting into this journey, you are taking the first step toward opting out of the cheap, insulting lies you've been fed by a system that is here to pimp you out for profits. It might take a while to get there, and that's OK. It took a while to get where you are today. We'll take it one step at a time—in sisterhood.

FROM FALSE SELF-CARE TO SOUL CARE

As a mother of a daughter, and as a psychologist who specializes in supporting women, my deepest desire is that you abandon the belief that there was ever anything wrong with you, and that you lean fully into this single truth: You are, and have always been, a miracle.

We discussed seeking sisterhood and the pervasiveness of toxic beauty culture. Now let's start to explore the difference between false self-care and soul care.

Women have been programmed from a young age to spend time, money, and energy on our appearance. As teens, many of us went to tanning beds—something that feels unfathomable to me today! As young adults, we started dyeing our hair and going to nail appointments. As full-on adults, we have regular hair and nail appointments, and often facials and the occasional, well-timed touch-up Botox. It may not surprise you to learn that researchers have found that the more someone uses social media, the more time they spend on beauty enhancement.[7]

I say: enough. Now, I'm not suggesting that we reject beauty. But you can feel beautiful without doing so from a place of seeking worthiness.

If you choose to stick with me through this entire book, my deepest hope is that you fully understand the magnificence of aging and the profound experience of womanhood. That you're able to meet the little girl within you who still has big dreams and loves with her whole heart. After all, you're already undergoing a journey of uncovering deep authenticity and self-reverence just by reading this sentence. Continuing with this book is another step down the path I'm offering: an alternative to fear.

My hope is simply that you're starting to ask questions now. That something primal has been stirred in you, a fury for being under a spell for so long. Maybe you're not sure how you feel yet, and that's OK. It can take time to fully uncover, and make sense of, the alternate reality you've been living in. By the end of our journey together in this book, you will begin to excavate for the truth of your heart and access your ancient wisdom. You will begin to rediscover, and fully reconnect with, your power. And you will understand that everything you ever needed already resides inside you.

I want this book to feel like retracing your steps into the bountiful woods of childlike self-wonder. We'll take a walk together, back to the little girl version of you, the one who was left behind, the one whose dreams were scattered in the dust and nearly lost. The little girl who abandoned herself when the brainwashing began. The version of you whose huge dreams, vulnerable heart, and admiration for herself were traded for the version of you the world wanted: pretty, small, pleasing, quiet.

Through the pages of this book, I'll walk you step-by-step through uncovering what is and crafting what can be. This isn't a simple framework to apply—1, 2, 3, and, poof, you're magically healed. Rather, it's a radical reorienting that begins a lifetime of change. Importantly, we will explore the reality of the world we live in and the world we create within ourselves, and I'll provide specific activities throughout this book for you to engage in. Along the way, I'll share stories, case studies, data, and personal experience to deepen learning.

You can engage in this book in whatever way feels right to you. You might be at a stage where all you can do is read and think, and that's OK. But if you want the full experience, I invite you to try the activities I share— from rewriting your beliefs to rage-release practices to cultivating pleasure. I've brought my knowledge from decades as a psychologist to support you on this journey.

It will take time to journey to revolutionary womanhood, but if you stick with it, you'll get there. Be patient with yourself. After all, most of us have been running in the opposite direction our entire lives. As I mentioned in the introduction, the average girl realizes around the tender age of nine years old that the most valuable thing she has to offer is her beauty. She spends the rest of her life contorting, starving, silencing, and complying so she can feel loved, chosen, and approved of. Her big dreams get traded for conformity.

When millions of us begin to wake up and demand something better, we do so for generations of women who have been silenced. I want to be on the front lines of calling out the disease of being youth obsessed. The sickness in selling the message of preventative Botox to twenty-year-old girls, the fearmongering that begins before she even starts living.

This book will most likely stir an inferno either way. You'll either feel anger toward a system that has duped us all . . . or you will feel irritated that this information has even been brought to your consciousness. If you decide to continue this journey with me, you'll be forced to confront and undo deeply held beliefs about your inadequacy and push back against an entire culture that wants to keep you down. Of course, you can ignore what I'm sharing and continue to live in submission to the world that multibillion-dollar corporations have created. Or you can recognize the reality of this world and choose to reject their messages and live fully. Either way, there will be a stirring. Such self-examination is too personal for it to not be jarring. You must make an active decision to be conscious of, or submissive to, the war on women. And at the heart of this exploration, you must ask the question: How will I allow my life to be written? The choices are patriarchal fear or matriarchal truth.

I want a better, more beautiful story for us—and for the millions of sisters following behind us. We get to tell a different story, for all of us, so that someday we may all be free.

To fully understand how we became so far removed from our ancient feminine leadership and intuition, we must first look at how history has shaped the narrative. Let's begin by examining how we even got here.

Chapter 2

THE HISTORY OF WHY WE ARE HERE

"Peace in patriarchy is war against women."

—MARIA MIES, *PATRIARCHY AND ACCUMULATION ON A WORLD SCALE*

IN 1998, MELBOURNE, Australia's Professor Helen O'Connell diagramed and detailed the full anatomy of the clitoris, changing women's health care, medical anatomy books, and female sexual satisfaction forever. Her work also illuminates a pervasive core of patriarchy: fear, lack of understanding, and even erasure of the female body and sexuality.

Let's not skim over the date this work began. Note that Dr. O'Connell published her work just a couple of decades ago. That means medical professionals didn't have access to accurate anatomical information about a woman's clitoris until 1998. The same medical professionals who were supposed to care for women's bodies didn't even know where a key part of it was.

O'Connell wanted to change that. Her quest began as a medical student, when she read the book *Last's Anatomy* to prepare for her surgical exam. In an interview for *The Sydney Morning Herald*, she called this "the ridiculous book" because it barely mentioned the clitoris and didn't include any illustrations. The textbook even referred to female genitalia as a "failure" of male genital formation. How was she supposed to prepare for her future patients if her medical studies didn't include a full education on the vulva? There were, however, two entire pages dedicated to the penis.

The textbook wasn't a one-off. A study examining anatomy texts studied by students in the US published in 1992 in the journal *Social Science & Medicine* showed that "[in] illustrations, vocabulary and syntax, these texts primarily depict male anatomy as the norm or standard against which female structures are compared." The researchers add that modern medical textbooks of the day were still influenced by "long-standing historical conventions in which male anatomy provides the basic model for 'the' human body."[1]

Thankfully, O'Connell wasn't one to accept the status quo. When she was twenty-seven, she read the book *A New View of a Woman's Body* by the Federation of Feminist Women's Health Centers in the United States and instantly knew this information had to be brought to the wider medical world. The book contained illustrations of vulvas, drawn with great detail—and yes, including the clitoris. The researchers gave this special organ specific attention in an entire chapter detailing their findings. To learn about the clitoris, the researchers undressed from the waist down, comparing their vulvas with the illustrations in reputable medical anatomy books. Then they did something controversial: They took turns masturbating, studied each other's orgasms, and documented the clitoris's role in sexual pleasure, as well as how it changed during the process.

While O'Connell found their information intriguing and valid, she also knew it wasn't conducted in a way that would be accepted by the medical community. And she knew she needed to be the one to change that.

BECOMING "CLITERATE" AFTER YEARS OF MALE-FOCUSED TEXTBOOKS

At the time, she was studying her master's of medicine in women's health at the University of Melbourne, which meant she had access to cadavers and a lab. "We just needed to do good science and work it out from the cadavers," she told *The Sydney Morning Herald*.[2]

Her specific area of focus: the clitoral bulbs. Even as late as the 1990s, medical anatomy books usually left out this important part of the clitoris. Not only did they omit the fact that the bulbs become engorged during arousal, but if they were included at all, they were normally drawn in the wrong place, much smaller than would be anatomically correct, and labeled "bulbs of the vestibule." In medicine, a vestibule refers to a cavity that opens to another entrance—so this was about as ambiguous a description as researchers could assign.

Chances are you don't know what a clitoral bulb is either—even in modern times, many of us aren't educated on the anatomy of the vulva. For context, the clitoral bulbs are located along either side of the urethra, extending between the head of the clitoris and the vagina.

This was careless medicine and Dr. O'Connell would prove to be up to the task of righting these anatomically incorrect wrongs. She gathered her team, procured ten cadavers, and dissected the pubic bone so she could see the inside of the clitoris. They took pictures and tested the tissues, carefully recording their findings. In 2005, O'Connell confirmed her original research with magnetic resonance imaging (MRI). She studied ten women, whose clitorises lit up vibrantly in the imaging because of the high blood flow.

She later published her findings in a paper titled "Anatomy of the Clitoris" in *The Journal of Urology*, detailing the anatomical structure of the clitoris, including the bulbs. The paper includes real pictures of dissected clitorises, MRI scans, and detailed illustrations of the various components of the clitoris. She discusses not only form but function, and she details how medicine's understanding of the female body has been impacted by social influences rather than anatomical facts. She also calls out the imbalance in representation of men's and women's sexual organs in medical texts.[3]

Not only did O'Connell become Australia's first female urologist, but her work changed the medical landscape globally. It shifted how doctors understood and treated women's reproductive and urologic organs, including improving surgical techniques used during pelvic surgery to protect patients' sexual sensation. And it transformed how we as women understand our own bodies.[4] Importantly, her work has inspired continued research: A quick search on Google Scholar for "clitoris orgasm" shows 2,520 studies published since 2022.[5]

And on that note, the orgasms rate is abysmal for women compared with men. In 2015, *Psychology Today* published an article on "the orgasm gap." One study of 15,000 people ages eighteen to sixty-five found that when two people who are familiar with each other have sex, heterosexual women have orgasms only 63 percent of time compared with 85 percent of heterosexual or gay men.[6] Understanding the clitoris is one step toward understanding female pleasure.

But while her impact has been great, our medical understanding—and treatment of—women's bodies still has a lot of room for medical innovation. In this chapter, we'll dig deeper into this history through an exploration of medicine, law, and cinema. We'll explore how little women are valued, as evidenced by a lack of innovation across industries, and how patriarchy has been intentionally built to control women. Understanding the history is foundational to undoing the shackles of patriarchy and beginning to shape a brighter future: one anchored in matriarchy.

THE MEDICAL MALPRACTICE OF MARKETING FEAR

It's true there has been medical advancement and modernization in almost every field of medicine, including women's health, thanks to pioneers like

Dr. O'Connell. Tools and devices for both daily procedures and surgeries are constantly being reimagined and designed for comfort, effectiveness, and safety. But it is important to note that one particular annual procedure for women that brings in billions of dollars in revenue globally has made little advancement: pap smears. One medical device, the pap smear speculum, is still being used in close to its original form from the 1800s.[7]

It's important to understand the history of James Marion Sims, once touted as "the father of gynecology," who designed this tool. He experimented on enslaved women, performing painful surgeries on them without administering anesthesia—operating on one woman, known only as Anarcha, thirty times.[8] Later, in his autobiography, which was published posthumously, he expressed his hatred for exploring the organs within the female pelvis.[9] In 2018, Sims's statue was removed from New York's Central Park because he is considered a controversial figure.[10]

So one of our most important health devices was invented by a torturer with disdain for the very procedure he invented. No wonder the speculum is hauntingly barbaric.

While some modifications have been made to the original speculum, the design has essentially stayed the same. Some companies—including Yona, FemSuite, and Doctor's Research Group Inc.—have tried to innovate and get a better speculum to market, but most medical offices still use an archaic form of this device,[11] and their work has largely been rejected by physicians.[12] One company, Nella, brought a more comfortable speculum to the market in 2020. But as of this writing, it's being marketed to women to bring to their own appointments. While I'm sure the company is making big efforts to get their product into health centers around the country, and I commend their efforts, I find it sad that women have to buy their own health-care kits, and bring them along to their appointments so they can suffer less. This is yet another way in which women's health and comfort is not valued.

Or consider the mammogram: In order to check for potential breast cancer, women need to have their breasts smashed between plates and be exposed to low X-ray radiation. Or the IUD, which I've heard described as excruciatingly painful and traumatizing. Or other forms of birth control like the pill, which might not physically hurt but can cause lifelong hormonal problems and a risk of blood clots, which can cause death. Or that the first known study on the absorbency of menstrual products using real blood—not a saline mixture—was published in 2023. You read that right: 2023.[13]

Many female doctors agree that the system is flawed when it comes to treating women's bodies, especially as they age. I interviewed two ob-gyns on my podcast, both from different medical schools and generations—one in her late forties, the other almost seventy—and each held a similar perspective. They shared that during their gynecological studies and rotations, there was little information or education on a woman's body after the age of thirty-five. It was as if, after the peak of her fertility years, a woman was no longer of use and therefore there was nothing to teach the students. Only after they reached midlife themselves did these two women doctors come to understand the massive void in the medical system, and both have gone on to open menopause-specific clinics for the gynecological needs of older women. And because they weren't able to find continuing education classes, they had to do extensive self-study to be able to adequately care for their patients.

It is imperative to educate ourselves about our bodies and our options. We must approach more of our lives—including medical procedures—from a place of informed choice instead of leaving decisions in the hands of others. Learned helplessness is a conditioned response. We have been taught to believe that we do not know, we are not capable, the doctor knows better. Passivity never creates a feeling of power. Rather, quite the opposite.

It's clear that women's bodies, health, and sexuality have been dangerously misrepresented, misunderstood, and mistreated, but the question remains: *Why?* Why has there been limited medical advancement in female health care? Why have we as women not loudly voiced our concerns? Why do we accept what is and not ask for better? Why do we not demand more?

Why have medical professionals not adopted a more humane, comfortable speculum? And what about the mammogram—does it get any more barbaric than this machine that smashes the breasts like pancakes? It's unlikely men would tolerate a machine that smashed their testicles into discs. So why do we as women continue to stay quiet about these torture devices? And why is it taking so long for a men's birth control to make it to the market—one that men will actually use? Why should we be the ones to suffer the side effects of birth control when we aren't even having as many orgasms *and* often experience the pain of childbirth?

Our silence is our vote for the medical system to stay the same. When we do not speak out about the imbalance in power—when we accept it and stay complicit—we are perpetuating the sexism that pervades every aspect of a woman's life.

But still, the question remains: Why? To begin to answer that question, we have to look back thousands of years.

> *Our silence is our vote for the medical system to stay the same. When we do not speak out about the imbalance in power—when we accept it and stay complicit—we are perpetuating the sexism that pervades every aspect of a woman's life.*

CENTURIES OF LEGALLY SUBORDINATING WOMEN

In the book *Creation of Patriarchy*, Gerda Lerner explores how women have been subordinated over the centuries through the deliberate creation and structure of patriarchy. Lerner discusses how, as laws evolved and religions grew, women's inferior position in society further deteriorated. They were kept away from intellectual pursuits. Women's access to learning and religion was increasingly reduced—until they were eventually cut off from all sources of history-making.

A disturbing revelation of the book is that men learned and perfected cultural dominance by practicing it on women. They exerted control over them. Women were considered "things" more than "human beings" and were traded as a commodity, marking the beginning of women's subordination. Women were also regarded as diseased or abnormal in relation to menstruation, pregnancy, and menopause, and thus considered the inferior sex.

All of this female subjugation was done legally, with the blessing of both the courts and broader society. And yet there was no route for women to break free, to chart their own paths, or to stand in their own power. Men had social mobility based on the simple fact that they were male, and they could establish class or transcend it based on their economic success. Women's class and worth, on the other hand, were always determined by their sexual ties to a man.

For example, veiling of women began in the second millennium BCE in Mesopotamia as an effort to segregate women into the categories of respectable and disrespectable women. Guess what established respectability? Marriage. The respectable woman—married woman—had to be veiled, while women who weren't married could not wear a veil; and it was also written into law that it was the duty of citizens to report women who went against these norms. An enslaved girl who was caught wearing a veil was subject to severe punishment, often by having her clothes taken away and cutting her ears off. Because wearing a veil in public became a symbol of status, married women bought into this norm and complied. Women's class status came to be defined by their relationship to men, while men were defined by their contribution to the economic system, and the separation between what elevates women and men in societal class remains today.

Lerner also details the removal of the goddesses from mainstream religion. Goddess worship—honoring the sacredness of female sexuality and its mysterious life-giving force, which included the power to heal—was prevalent in one form or another throughout the ancient world. The rise of Abrahamic religions, however, led to the erasure of the goddess. Simultaneously, woman came to be seen as the omen of death and sin in the world. Through law and religion, women's sexuality came to be linked with sin and temptation. Enter: the veil.

From life-giving source of the universe and healer to sinful and dangerous—such a devastating fall from grace. All done in the name of controlling women.

As focus shifted from powerful goddesses to a single male god, women were further erased in religion. These developments coincided with more marginalization of women. Males alone could be mediators between god and man while women were denied equal access to learning, lawmaking, and priesthood. Women were no longer seen as having the capacity for interpreting and altering religious belief systems.

In nearly every aspect of human life, women have been controlled by men—stripped of power and autonomy over even our own bodies. We were historically deprived of receiving education, and removed from leadership in religion, art, law, medicine, philosophy, and science. History was written and directed by men, and women were merely there to serve in support roles. When women are removed as storytellers, lawmakers, philosophers, religious leaders, and decision-makers, society is not balanced. There is no room for honoring our half of humanity through this half-told creation and history.

Without significant contributions by women in medicine, science, philosophy, and other critical fields, we will pass on to the next generations the same imbalance. Even as I write this, history seems to be perpetuating itself in relation to women's reproductive rights in the United States. As American women start to reclaim our voices and power, and step more into politics and leadership, the legal system is moving backward, trying to take our inherent rights away—including access to abortion and even contraception.

History influences how we understand our identity and relate to the world. Medicine, law, and entrepreneurship are examples of how our history has been defined by the patriarchy. If history continues to be shaped by men, we will forever be stuck on the carousel of imbalance.

ARISTOTLE'S TROUBLING VIEW OF WOMEN

When history has been written and informed by men, told from only one-half of our societal story, it's no wonder we as women have formed our identities from this male perspective. We've viewed ourselves, our roles, and our feelings in relation to the patriarchal checklist—a man's definition of a good woman. We've been regularly referred to as the inferior sex, subservient, weak, and hysterical, with limited contributions to philosophy, law, art, or science; it makes sense that we would see ourselves as unworthy, feeling second-class to men.

Consider the perspectives of Aristotle, who is widely considered one of the world's greatest thinkers and philosophers. In *Politics*, Aristotle declares that "there are by nature various classes of rulers and ruled. For the free rules the slave, the male the female, and the man the child in a different way." Men, he explains, hold greater morality and virtue; he goes on to write that "the poet said of woman: 'Silence gives grace to woman—' though that is not the case likewise with a man."[14]

In another work, *On the Generation of Animals*, he writes that "the female is as it were a deformed male; and the menstrual discharge is semen, though in an impure condition; i.e., it lacks one constituent, and one only, the principle of Soul."[15]

Consider this: Because Aristotle is one of our most revered thought leaders, future thought leaders have built upon his precepts. Entire college courses are dedicated to his work. When one of the most revered thinkers in history sees women as biologically and morally inferior, how might his influence show up in our broader systems, including medicine, law, and entertainment?

Until now, only a partial, distorted record has been told—and from the male viewpoint only, with the male as the superior star. As we've explored, even women's health has made very few advancements. In fact, most everything we relate to as women has been based on what men have created: yoga, meditation, exercise, calorie intake, movies, music, comedy, art, medical procedures. Of course we feel like something is missing!

Some of these are even marketed to us under the guise of female empowerment.

Ah, there's a word I don't love: empowerment. Let's unpack that concept.

The work of empowerment has been primarily focused on women. But consider this: It is rare for men to speak of becoming more empowered. Even the word "empowerment" has a flavor of asking for permission. Of waiting for power to be granted. I call bullshit on this. Women want power over their bodies, their voice, their choices, their careers, and their relationships. And we can find that agency ourselves—we don't need someone else to grant us the right to rule our own lives.

But most of us are too afraid to fully step into power because it comes with a cost. After all, we've seen what happens to powerful women. They're judged and vilified. They're whispered about. They're held to impossible standards. They're called a bitch. And often, other women deliver these punishments. No wonder we're afraid.

Women have feared power primarily because of how it has been used—disproportionately and dangerously exploited in the hands of men throughout history. Most men seek power *over* while most women seek power *within*, and these are very different approaches and energies. The differentiator here is that most women are communal and collaborative. But if we cannot claim and hold our own power, then we essentially have zero agency and will forever ricochet around, bouncing between other people's choices for our lives. It's critical for women to step into personal power in all aspects of their lives. We need more women leading and teaching the masses how to be powerful, in a deeply integrated way.

In order to access power in your own life, the first step is an internal examination of the story you have been operating by when you think of women in power. Do you feel threatened, intimidated, or triggered? Or do you wish to be bold, clear, and powerful? In either case, where did you learn to feel this way?

You must also actively make space for other powerful women. As the saying goes, "a rising tide lifts all boats." This is the journey we are taking together in this book: tapping into your inner power—the power that has always been there, waiting to be claimed. And we're also tapping into our collective female power, helping other women rise as we rise ourselves.

Additionally, we have to get raw and honest about our own participation in the system. We cannot simply point our fingers outward, blaming everyone but ourselves. The work of undoing centuries of subjugation starts with a single woman: you.

HISTORY IS ONLY HALF THE STORY

How have we as women been complicit in this half-written history? If you look at the word "history," it literally reads *his* story. The etymology of the word is from Greek *histōr*, meaning "learned wise man."[16] It's important to note that history is both what has happened and also what is happening, because we are influencing history every second of every day.

When we come into consciousness about the fact we have been living and functioning with only half the story, we must allow this knowing to become the force that moves us into action and to change how we navigate within a male-dominated society. We cannot create change from a limited mindset, a half-told history, and a resignation that this is how it has always been and we have no power to effect change.

Instead, we must counter this skewed narrative with honesty. We must anchor to a mindset rooted in what feels aligned and true and reject the storyline of expectations that have been passed down from a patriarchal context—stories that intend to control and placate.

Yet so much of what women believe about themselves is based on a deeply flawed system. Even in modern times, we are deeply influenced by the stories of men, especially in the cinema. This lack of female narratives is why I've never been a movie fan—I find most of them to be grotesquely violent, and I typically walk away feeling deeply unsatisfied, even after watching the so-called love stories. I crave more nuanced characters and deeper pursuits of human connection.

Several years ago, I found myself begrudgingly sitting next to my husband and kids in the theater, all of them thrilled to watch an action movie that had just been released. I kept telling myself to be a "good sport" for the sake of their excitement, even wondering why I could not just chill out a bit and not take everything so seriously. But deep down, the self-talk felt inauthentic. As the movie began, I willed myself to find the entertainment in it. But only fifteen minutes in, I felt a hot rage that I could no longer ignore. The violent, gory visuals and human brutality upset my whole nervous system. To sit there any longer was a massive betrayal of myself. I leaned over and told my family that I would be outside waiting for them when the movie was over.

After quickly exiting the darkened theater, I immediately walked to the building exit and went for a long walk. I was furious. How in the hell was watching people shoot each other considered entertainment? All I felt was disgust.

My reaction that day was cumulative. For a couple of years, I had been in conscious awareness of my feelings during and after movies. And not just while watching action movies but also love stories, documentaries, and comedies. Later, I did a brief online search and discovered the disconnect for me: Most movies are directed by men! A staggering 10.1 men are hired for every 1 female director in fictional films—meaning 91 percent of fictional movies are directed by men, and an oddly parallel 91 percent of movies contain violence, some with extreme violence.[17] These statistics explained it all for me. I felt sane. Validated. In that moment, I realized that stories told through the lens of men represented only half of the story. No wonder I longed for so much more.

There are so few female directors telling the stories of our hearts, our perspectives, our experiences. My discomfort and disgust signaled a deeper craving to see more of myself and my sisters represented on the screen. We are still viewing the world through the lens of patriarchy instead of matriarchy, even in the movies! And this male-centered mindset continues to be perpetuated by the men producing movies. The screen holds their interpretation of social roles, of love, of women's bodies. Men are defining humanity for us, and we're told to accept it as reality. Additionally, when a strong female is showcased in action movies, she's often dressed provocatively and shown to be physically strong and able to fight. There are minimal roles where strong women are not sexualized or masculine. And even when the stories feel wrong to us as women, it's hard to pinpoint the source of our discomfort. After all, what alternative do we have to compare these shows and movies to?

THE MALE PERSPECTIVE AS DEFAULT MODE

Men's interpretation of life is the dominant narrative, and, as such, it is what we as a society absorb and rarely question. These types of movies have been playing for so long that this one-sided narrative feels normal. We unconsciously accept that this is just the way it is, but deep down, we know something isn't right. You can begin to see the danger and conditioning that continues to be perpetuated in medicine, lawmaking, and Hollywood. We are like fish that don't know they're swimming around in patriarchal water. The male perspective is so insidious that we do not even question it—and that is why I felt so profoundly called to write this book for you.

Without context and research, it's difficult to consciously perceive the most obvious and important realities around us. And we can't understand where our society went wrong unless we look at both history and modernity.

Consider how most women have no problem learning from men—reading their books, listening to their music, attending their concerts, seeking them as mentors, healers, doctors, and gurus. Inversely, how many men do you know that take trainings from women, read books written by women, have playlists filled with female artists, and attend concerts of those female artists with their guy friends? How many men do you know who have a female mentor or healer? You can see how deeply this narrative runs for all of us.

Or take language nuance. How many times have you been in a group of people and someone said something like, "OK, guys, let's go," and you thought absolutely nothing of it. Now how many times has the mixed group been referred to as girls, as in, "OK, girls, let's go." I would imagine next to never, unless it was said in jest. The default sex is men, and while we may want to delude ourselves and say words are just words, the human experience is not that simple. Language impacts perception and behavior.

As we've explored, the storyline for what we perceive as ideal beauty, what seems reasonable for medical procedures, and absolutely everything else we experience in our daily lives as women is being informed through the lens of men. We consume and self-define from a male perspective, squeezing ourselves into compression clothing and slinking into thong bathing suits. We make major decisions about our lives based on standards written by men. We hide our gray hair and rounded bellies.

Can you begin to see how absolutely absurd this is? How little we have allowed women's voices to shape the landscape of our world? So many women are completely unconscious of their own womanhood being defined through the lens of patriarchy that they do not even question the rules of engagement.

BARBIE, THE MOVIE, FLIPS PATRIARCHY

And then came *Barbie*. In the summer of 2023, the blockbuster movie came to the big screen and grossed over $1.38 billion, becoming the highest-grossing film in the history of Warner Bros. Entertainment's one hundred years of making films.[18] It was a worldwide phenomenon and had everyone talking.

Without spoiling the movie, here's the basic plot. Barbie Land is a place where Barbies of all kinds—all with the same name of Barbie—live in complete harmony. Women hold all meaningful roles, including doctors, leaders, and politicians, including the country's president. Ken, again with the same name for all men, has value only when Barbie looks at him. His life is spent trying to get Barbie's approval so he can feel seen and validated. He dances, dotes, and smiles, hoping Barbie will give him attention. Eventually, Ken recognizes the imbalance and seeks to take male control over Barbie Land. If you haven't seen it, you'll have to watch the movie to find out what happens next.

For many, the film was the first time they recognized the effects of patriarchy. Gender imbalance became an issue only when the tables were completely turned and women were in control of everything. While many moviegoers felt validated, others were outraged. How dare Hollywood suggest that men actually rule the world and women don't have equal rights! Religious groups warned that *Barbie* was a brainwashing stunt and strongly advised people to not see it.

I wasn't surprised to see that the film wasn't given its due praise at the Oscars. Actor Ryan Gosling, who plays Ken, received an Oscar nomination for best actor, while Margot Robbie, who plays Barbie, and Greta Gerwig, the director, didn't receive nominations for their individual categories. And while the movie received nominations across eight categories, including best picture, it only won best song.

Snubs aside, the movie brilliantly illustrates how patriarchy controls the narrative and impacts women psychologically. While most people went to the theater with the intention of being entertained, many quickly realized the much deeper meaning as the story unfolded. As the inverted power dynamic and unjust treatment of the Kens played out on the big screen, it became nearly impossible to deny who *really* controls the world (men!), and how unbalanced our society really is.

After the movie, my twenty-year-old daughter said to me, "I found myself feeling bad for the Kens and how little control they had. And then I realized: Oh my gosh, this is how we as women live every single day. This is our actual reality.'"

The same was true for my clients. All around the world, client after client saw the movie, and the reactions were unanimous. So much sadness, outrage, anger, frustration, and overwhelm. Most women shared that they cried multiple times during the movie and left the theater with a heaviness in their hearts. I spoke with dozens of young women in their early twenties, many who had gone to the movie multiple times and then had discussion groups with their friends afterward. They shared how, for the first time, their daily realities felt validated. Many said their boyfriends, brothers, and fathers were finally able to somewhat understand what they had been trying to describe all along: the reality of being a female in a patriarchal world.

After speaking to countless women, from all age ranges, religions, and backgrounds, what I find most fascinating is that women want respect and equal power. They don't want power *over* another person, they want power over themselves, over their choices and bodies. Women want more professional opportunities. More gender-balanced child-rearing. Women want to feel safe when they walk down the street alone at night. They don't want to feel constantly gawked at and objectified. Women desire more balance in the societal system and structures.

The lack of consideration around our voices is infuriating and it perpetuates a highly dysfunctional system. As the feminist author and activist Caroline Criado Perez explains in her book *Invisible Women: Exposing Data Bias in a World Designed for Men*, when the female half of humanity is left out of system design, women are the ones who suffer in time, health, and money.[19]

Also worth noting, in addition to the *Barbie* movie, that same year the Taylor Swift and Beyoncé tours brought in unprecedented crowds, with never-before-seen numbers and women gathering in droves. An article in *Time* magazine titled "The Staggering Economic Impact of Taylor Swift's Eras Tour" said that Swift's US tour was projected to result in nearly $5 billion in consumer spending. Her tour made an estimated $4.1 billion, according to the *Washington Post*.[20] Beyoncé performed for 2.7 million fans in thirty-nine cities for her Renaissance World Tour; *Forbes* published a piece detailing how she pulled in a one-month gross revenue of $179.3 million—the highest of all musical artists, ever.[21]

These examples show there's a huge desire to connect with female power, to hear stories by women for women, and to celebrate being a woman.

So, the question becomes: Now what?

Where do we go from here?

How do we effect change?

How do we reimagine womanhood, for ourselves and for the collective?

PERFORMING FOR PATRIARCHY

As women struggle to gain "equal" roles in society, it becomes clear that the gains we've made are not enough. Men still ultimately control which women will get which roles, and they punish and ostracize those who attempt to challenge or rewrite the narratives.

So, what needs to happen for real change to take place in the societal system? We cannot continue trying to add a few women into a dysfunctional system, as that won't create actual change. To achieve a true paradigm shift, we must place women and children at the center of our societal system. From there, we will be able to dismantle patriarchy and create a more balanced way of life, power, respect, and control.

Patriarchy, after all, is a historical construct built to control women. To see significant change, we will need to begin the work of deconstructing it from the center—and rebuild it with a new model: matriarchy. Matriarchy is a system of society or government ruled by women.

This will be nearly impossible as long as women continue to expend significant energy on their looks. Female fixation on beauty, thinness, and antiaging are distractions that keep women focused on matters of the body rather than matters of the soul. Let me further break this down. Most women do not even realize that they are playing into, and feeding, the patriarchal beast by filling up their days with "maintenance" appointments. But the only thing being maintained is the storyline that women serve as objects, and that in order to "maintain" any relevance to men they must "maintain" a certain beauty standard. So, while women continue to squander their resources of time, money, and energy, they are complicit in a system that has no real desire to see women rise to power. So seduced by the empty promise of external measures being the most coveted, these women are exactly where the patriarchy wants them: brainwashed.

Such a shallow existence and pursuit! Women are still perpetuating the storyline that one's only real value is in her flawless appearance, her ability to please men, and her eternal youth. This is a deeply sick mindset that has no soulful destination; it's allowing oneself to serve as a function rather than a human. It does not contribute to change for the female collective and our future as women.

We may think we're fighting for our place, but make no mistake, the masses of women are still trying to advance within the patriarchal lens. Just look around. Examples are everywhere of the performative feminine as opposed to rooted feminine, which we will explore further in coming chapters. There is nothing deeply rooted or powerful about freezing your face with fillers or Botox. Instead, such self-harm indicates the terror of no longer being relevant. Of becoming invisible.

After all, this invisible older woman is a story the world knows all too well. Men are revered for their sexy gray hair and wrinkles while women are punished for showing a single sign of aging. We lose jobs and partners. And nothing will change if we continue to play the game and feed into this vicious, never-ending loop.

Look at the way we treat our bodies. From a spiritual perspective, when women inject toxins into their forehead in an effort to hide the dreadful "eleven lines" between the eyes, they are freezing their third eye chakra and disconnecting from their intuition, their energy source. The disturbing culture of women looking like mannequins sets us tragically far back as women. There is nothing enlightened or advancing for us if we pump our faces full of toxins. It is deeply desperate, and we are complicit to the story that aging is a failure, and only youthful women are worthy. And as women continue to punish themselves by starving, endless dieting, and punishing workouts, they play into the story that women who take up less space are more valuable. As women continue to stuff their bodies into shapewear, they not only harm their internal organs and digestion but disconnect from and torture their womb space, the most powerful portal where endless inner wisdom resides.

Women participate in all of these games, performing for patriarchy, doing the dance of self-terrorism without looking up to realize they're nothing more than puppets on strings. These acts of self-harm are not anchored one ounce into the profound wisdom of the divine feminine. So while we may try to convince ourselves these choices come from a powerful place, at the root is terror and fear of becoming irrelevant, invisible, not chosen, unlovable. And as long as we continue to live by the most insulting rules for our existence, nothing will ever change.

It's on us women to change the fucking rules.

SHAME AND DISCONNECTION REPLACE FEMALE POWER

When Western civilization built the patriarchy, women were stripped of their rights, their power, their priesthood, their ministries, their voices, and their leadership. This caused a degradation of the rituals and practices women lived and led by, which were built on deep intuition. Women continued to lose more and more of their inherent rituals with each generation.

Women used to pass down rituals from their ancestors; now women pass down shame. Women used to commune; now women compete, another symptom of patriarchy. When there are fewer men to marry—to secure food, shelter, and safety—women are conditioned to compete for those positions. Now, in more modern times, when there are fewer seats at the board table, women step on one another to secure their spots. Yet shame and competition leave us feeling threatened and keep us so busy infighting that we will never become powerful enough to effect any great structural change for all women (and men).

And it's getting worse. With each passing generation, women further disconnect from their bodies and cycles. There is little to no deep connection around the most sacred parts of a woman's life: periods, childbirth, menopause.

Rather than honoring each cycle, it's becoming more routine to opt out of each phase—to numb, reverse, and medicate—all of which only serve to take us even further away from our intuition, our deep knowing. It makes sense that we have learned to hate and fear our own bodies: the chaos, mess, and inconvenience they bring. We have been brainwashed to believe our body cycles and natural phases are disgusting and we need to do something about the inconvenience.

Rather than seeing our womanhood as power, we seek to be more pleasing. More palatable. When men control the narrative—and when we never pause to question the author—we eventually lose our way completely. We get so far removed from our sacred connections that we begin to normalize the way we abandon our bodies. To support reconnection, we'll explore the female body in more depth later in the book.

There are so few stories passed down from our mothers and grand-mothers about the sacredness of womanhood: periods, birthing, menopause, and all of the beautiful physicality of being a woman. Stories connect us. We learn from them: about the women who went before us. About our sisters. About ourselves.

Instead of uplifting stories, we now have shame. We have disconnected completely from these holy rites of passage. The functioning of the female body is seen as a series of massive inconveniences that need to be managed and controlled rather than surrendered to. Without women passing down stories of power—stories filled with reverence and divinity—we get fur-ther away from any connection to this exquisite tapestry of womanhood. Women used to gather and honor each other during menstrual periods and home births. For example, the Karuk Tribe, located in California, have a coming-of-age ceremony when girls get their first periods.[22] Many more Indigenous tribes used to hold ceremonies—that is, until the male coloniz-ers began to rape the women, believing their dancing was a signal for them to be dominated.[23]

Women are suffering deeply. We are in a profound crisis. The feminine has been vilified, fracked, and far removed from holiness. We have been gaslit for so long that we do not even believe in or trust our own bodies. We chase outside approval and use the most insulting measures to determine our worthiness.

There is a core longing for community, gathering, rituals, and holiness. This desire is within every woman I speak to and work with. This longing is so inherent that many women go to church simply to feel the rituals and holiness. But the efforts we make to feel complete never last because they are patriarchal and external. They do not pierce at the level we crave, because what we actually crave is our own holiness, our own feminine ways of connecting that have nothing to do with religion but instead are anchored in a divinity inherent to being a woman.

Women are communal by nature and thrive in safe sisterhood. We are creators, healers, and magic makers for one another. We were never meant to do life alone. I believe much of the depression and loneliness women feel is because they have become so disconnected, isolated from any form of tribe or sisterhood.

We can't look to the patriarchy for answers. As Audre Lorde said, "The master's tools cannot dismantle the master's house."[24] Your path forward must be both internal and communal. And it will feel revolutionary.

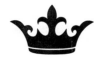

Section II

IDENTIFY
THE SYSTEMS

Chapter 3

THE JOURNEY TO REVOLUTIONARY WOMANHOOD

"The body, like everything else in life, is a mirror of our inner thoughts and beliefs. Every cell within your body responds to every single thought you think and every word you speak."

—LOUISE HAY, *LOVE YOUR BODY*

LET US BEGIN by imagining the unimaginable. A world where women are no longer at war with themselves. Envision a reality in which women consider their looks and body shape to be the least interesting things about them. In which women spend their money in ways that expand and enhance their souls rather than on products and procedures that disguise their perceived flaws. In which med spas are replaced with sanctuaries that offer sacred mirror rituals, sensual dancing, rage-release practices, and ancient rites of passage ceremonies.

Picture a society in which women nourish and replenish from within. In which they care more for their spirit than their faces. In which women are deeply connected to their inherent worthiness and spend time honoring their natural cycles, rather than seeing female bodies as inconvenient and something to apologize for. They see their bodies as temples—which they would never disparage or desecrate but instead tend by breathing pleasure and love into them. A world where women stop explaining themselves and looking for approval. Where they are no longer objectified by men or treated as second-class citizens.

A world where women are safe. Celebrated. Just as they are.

Now imagine yourself in that space: loved, whole, seen.

This is a reality I am already living. I am here to show you the way to that world, just as I have with my clients. Living this way is possible and it begins within you. You have to decide you will be the change. There is no waiting for a fairy godmother to bestow a new life upon you. It's yours for the creating.

CHANGE HAS TO START WITH US

We women must be the ones to create that new reality, because the only way the patriarchal status quo will ever change is by each of us changing it. We enact change by creating new expectations and standards for our lives—for our relationships, our careers, our bodies, our roles in society. Left to the patriarchy to "fix" these things, nothing will change.

We've explored that history has been written by men and for men. Almost every war, school shooting, rape, molestation, and genocide has occurred at the hands of men. Greed. Power. Ego. Each fuels these never-ending atrocities. Patriarchy is controlling and requires domination over others. It destroys and traumatizes.

Matriarchy, on the other hand, is collaborative, communal, and solutions-based. It nourishes, guides, and heals. Women intuitively lead with compassion and an innate caring for humanity and the planet.

In this moment as our world burns and endless, unspeakable atrocities continue to rise, we must take stock of what we believe and examine our internal guidance system, which leads us when we make decisions about our lives and the people we love.

As you observe the state of the world, does it appear men are prioritizing women and protecting them? Or does it appear there is an agenda based on control? The patriarchy hurts everyone, men included. The system does not raise men to be in their divine masculine. Rather, they are raised to toughen up and not express emotions. This philosophy destroys us all. On the other hand, the divine masculine serves and protects us all—and not from a place of dominance or control over others.

Instead of anchored decision-making, I find most people are on automatic pilot. Rarely, if ever, do individuals look at the root of their consciousness. I hope the ideas in this book push you to sit with, and understand, what you believe, and most importantly, why you believe it. This work can be uncomfortable, even triggering. It can feel enraging to realize how many thousands of years women have suffered under the patriarchy.

It's tempting to want to look away, to placate our discomfort through the endless distractions offered in our modern world: work, television, social media, maintenance appointments (Botox, nails, facials, etc.). But our children and future generations *need* us to be brave enough to begin doing this work. We are in a global crisis! Earth is getting hotter; people are forced to migrate to find work and feed their families; anti-immigration sentiment is on the rise; and human rights are being suppressed in developed and developing countries alike.

Women are often outraged at the devastation globally but feel powerless and distant from the problems of the world. Maybe you've felt this way too. As I suggest to my clients, if you want to be part of systemic change, you must first start with your own burning house. While it can feel reasonable to keep your eyes fixated outward, blaming bad leaders and misguided citizens, the work within your own walls is how change begins. And it's how you, along with other intentional women, effect generational change and collective impact.

Internal work is difficult. And it's deeply personal.

It's critical to recognize how female placidity is perpetuated. As we've discussed, most women experience womanhood through the lens of patriarchy. We think, believe, decide, spend, judge, and express ourselves within a system that was written to control and oppress us.

The majority of women I speak with tell me they can't make certain choices in their lives because a "good wife" wouldn't do so. Or because they believe their desires would be seen as selfish and greedy, a result of internalizing the virtue of selflessness. Or because they're afraid of how others would react to a change in their behavior.

Change starts with paying attention to the rules, stories, and expectations absorbed from our cultures, families, and religions. In this chapter, we'll journey side-by-side as you do the necessary work of examining and deconstructing your beliefs. By understanding the rules you operate by, you'll be able to rewrite your beliefs—and create a more meaningful and fulfilling life.

REWRITING YOUR BELIEFS

To begin to undo these often unconscious beliefs, I have my clients make an exhaustive list of all the things they were told about what it means to be a woman. This list should include attributes, expectations, and any other words and phrases that define womanhood for them. After the list is complete, I ask them to sit with each individual list item and examine whether it's a true personal belief or one that feels untrue and was inherited from the world. For many women, their definition of womanhood has become so interwoven and enmeshed internally that it feels hard to decipher what is actually their own. With effort, they can untangle what they hold true from what society wants them to believe but doesn't resonate with them.

From this awareness, I then ask them to replace the attributes they don't believe in with more beautiful ones that align with their inner beliefs.

For example, one client was taught by both her family and her religion that women should stay home and give up any career aspirations, as rearing children was a woman's primary role. She saw this being reinforced by nearly all of the women in her community. For many years, she didn't question this belief and followed what was expected of her.

When we started working together, she was profoundly unhappy. I always begin with belief systems, as this is often the root cause of all suffering. It's distressing to live under a set of inherited beliefs that do not truly align with who you are at your core. We discovered that she didn't believe a mother has to choose between having children and having a meaningful career. When she was able to replace that installed, faulty belief with one that felt truer for her, she was able to live a freer, happier, more aligned life—at work and at home.

Like this client when we first met, few women ever pause to identify and examine their beliefs. Few ask themselves: What beliefs influence how I'm building my life? Typically, women operate from a deeply flawed belief system. Think of it like an old computer processing system, one that is outdated, riddled with viruses, and ineffective. When you rewrite these faulty beliefs into new ones that align with your core values, it's like installing an updated, more compatible operating system on which you can build an anchored life.

This exercise of listing and examining beliefs is vital for you to complete, as it will help identify the beliefs you have been basing your life on. I suggest you pause your reading here, take out a piece of paper, and make your list. Include all the attributes you were taught make for a "good woman." Give yourself plenty of time to do this—at least thirty minutes—and even when you feel like you've made an exhaustive list, pause and check in with yourself. You might uncover something profound.

From here, do just as I instruct my clients. Examine each belief and ask yourself: Does this hold true for me? If not, how would I rewrite this belief?

As an example, consider the belief that being a good woman means staying in one's marriage no matter what, for the sake of the children. With this belief, a woman might allow verbal abuse, emotional disconnection, or worse. But if she starts to examine that belief and see it for what it is, she might ask herself: Do I actually believe that women must stay in a marriage no matter the circumstances? Would I want my daughter to stay in a toxic marriage? Do I truly believe staying married is the only option?

When this woman digs deep, she'll probably discover that she absorbed this belief from her family or religion, so much so that she thinks it's hers.

As you begin to notice the beliefs you have attached yourself to, you'll begin to see the ways in which your beliefs have informed your choices. You'll find them underpinning how you live, how you make decisions, and why you feel the way you do about your body, relationships, gender roles, sensuality, power, and other women. If you have been conditioned to believe you are only worthy of love if you are constantly serving others, or that your opinions are not as important as those of the men in your life, you will build a life of muted servitude. Over time, you'll not only grow resentful but also likely feel alone and unseen.

People are designed to need emotional intimacy. When someone builds a life deprioritizing that desire for connection, constantly pushing it away, they can end up seeking connection and being "seen" by having extramarital affairs. Behaviors like drinking, overeating, and excessive shopping can also creep in as ways to find fulfillment. But the chase and pursuit constantly leave one unsatisfied, unfulfilled, because these behaviors only serve to numb the deeper desire.

There is nothing humans desire more than being truly seen and loved, and yet most people spend their lives chasing connection without ever truly connecting, because we've never been taught how to construct a life of deep intimacy—including with ourselves.

The patriarchal guidelines, written by men to serve men, offer next to nothing when it comes to deep relational fulfillment, and these guidelines are the reason the majority of people deeply struggle to make meaning of their lives. This is why you must begin with understanding what you were taught to believe, and then sit with those beliefs to allow the truth—*your* truth—to percolate to the surface. For example, do you actually believe, deep in your bones, that only young women are beautiful? That as women age, they become disposable and irrelevant? Is that a belief that feels true inside of your womb space? Or were you conditioned by toxic beauty culture or your family to believe that only youth can be beautiful, so much so that you think it's your belief?

When doing this work, my clients often come into consciousness, sometimes for the very first time in their lives, and are shocked to discover that so much of their existence has been built on a belief system they were brainwashed into, not one that feels aligned and true for them. This exploration is the beginning of liberation, of curating a life that feels more magnificent and honoring.

EXAMINE THE MEANING

I question everything in my work and personal life, take nothing at face value, and seek to deeply understand the inner workings of my beliefs and that of my clients. This includes the meaning I assign to things. I believe meaning-making is an incredible female superpower, but one women rarely perform.

Alongside beliefs, meaning is another layer to understanding how you orient to the world. As an example, I had a client who believed her two divorces meant she was a failure at relationships. She bought into this self-concept so much that she allowed it to define and inform her life, including people-pleasing behavior toward her children, a fear of dating, and seeing herself as not worthy of love.

After getting to know her and seeing how much havoc this one faulty self-concept was wreaking on her life, I asked if she was willing to give a new meaning to her two divorces. Her curiosity was piqued, but she was highly skeptical. I then asked if it was possible that her two divorces meant she had experienced tremendous self-growth and had simply outgrown these relationships. That each relationship's ending was not a sign of failure but simply a change of course, a natural ending for two people who had walked as far as they could together. We looked at whether this meaning was truer and more expansive.

I then asked if she would be willing to try this new meaning on over the coming weeks and pay attention to how her body and soul felt. It turned out that not only did this meaning feel more aligned for her, it also allowed space for her relationship with her children to improve as she was no longer filled with guilt and the need to people please. She even created a dating profile because she was able to acknowledge that she was worthy and desired to meet someone.

All of these powerful shifts happened because she decided to assign new meaning to her two divorces. As my client discovered, we have incredible power to make exquisite meaning out of everything in our lives. Approaching life as a meaning-maker is an expansive mindset shift that will allow for more compassion, beauty, and love to flow into your life.

Using this same technique, ask yourself: What do I want to make being a woman mean?

I am no exception from these meaning-shifting experiences. As I've mentioned, I do this work myself, and one personal example stands out to me from many years ago. Every month, I would become extremely bloated during the days before my period, and I would make it mean that I looked awful and that my body was difficult to get into clothes. I dreaded this time of the month for decades.

After sitting with this feeling, I saw how destructive the meaning I had made was, and I decided to make my monthly bloat mean that my body was absolutely phenomenal. Every single month, I went through a powerful cycle and intricacies were happening in my womb. From this new meaning, I started treating myself differently.

Now, instead of disgust, I see a miracle. I am tender with myself. I use the heating pad, drink nourishing tea, and wear loose clothing. Not only do I no longer dread this time of month, but I also now commune with it, honor my body, and enjoy this more loving approach. And I have been able to raise my daughter to do the same for herself, as well as educate my sons and my husband as to what my body is experiencing. So not only have I been able to show up more beautifully for myself, but I have also been able to guide others about what one's monthly cycles mean and the power of a woman's body.

Another belief I used to hold was that my emotions were too much— too intense, too varied, too deep. I used to think that maybe there was something wrong with how much I felt. Why couldn't I just take things at face value like it seemed everyone else did, rather than feel the depths of most everything around me? A typical emotionally neutral day for most people was almost always a flood of emotions for me. I made myself wrong for a long time and wished I could just be more easygoing. That is, until I decided to rewrite what being emotional meant for me.

After spending time with this meaning, I realized that my ability to feel so much and so deeply is my superpower. My emotional depth is the quality that has allowed me to experience the absolute fullness and mystery of life. Every day feels like an adventure to me. I enjoy living fully into each moment! I'm here for such a short time, and I don't want to bypass an ounce of it. Since making this shift, I now hold deep reverence for my capacity to feel, and those who are in my life see this as my most beautiful quality.

Like in my examples, the meaning you assign to your experience as a woman can lead to limitless or limiting beliefs. When you shape meaning, you also impact your experience, behaviors, and relationships. As an active meaning-maker, it's important to understand that you are never the victim of your thoughts.

Let me say that again: You are *never* the victim of your thoughts.

You can change even the deepest-held meaning, the most limiting beliefs. However, change requires living differently. It necessitates being present in your life. You must be in observation of yourself and the meaning you assign, more curious than critical of your beliefs, and willing to craft a story that feels more nourishing, supportive, and luxurious.

Sometimes breaking up with limiting beliefs and suffering is a scary process. It begs the question: What will happen if I choose to be responsible for my thoughts? Who will I blame? Who will I become? Often, these shifts in mindset will require you to loosen the shackles of an identity that was built on suffering, and for many, unshackling feels like a free fall rather than freedom. I invite you to instead hold the possibility of radical responsibility as the beginning of living the most aligned and magical life. This has not only been my experience but also the experience of the majority of my clients. Some have described this kind of living like going from seeing the world in black-and-white

> *Sometimes breaking up with limiting beliefs and suffering is a scary process. It begs the question: What will happen if I choose to be responsible for my thoughts? Who will I blame? Who will I become?*

to stepping into the most bountiful land, full of technicolor and dimension beyond anything they'd ever experienced.

So, I'll ask you now: What meaning do you want to assign to being a woman? How do you want to experience womanhood? What beliefs do you want to anchor into around being a woman? These questions are crucial to explore and will bring you into a deeper connection with yourself. Write the answers in your journal and refer back to the list often, adding to it as you notice more of what you desire to feel. Being your own architect for a magical life begins with these questions. It starts with recognizing that you hold the power to assign meaning to absolutely everything.

Until you fully examine the meaning you assign, and the beliefs you hold, nothing will change. You're simply putting a bandage over the infection, replacing it daily so it doesn't ooze, so your wounds don't show. But you have to keep reapplying it. You have to keep doing the affirmations and all the bullshit that never really works, because you're not doing the deepest work of scooping out the infection and replacing it with beautiful healing.

The skill sets of self-awareness, meaning-making, and rewriting your beliefs will take your life from ordinary and mundane to feeling like a work of art, the most alluring movie, a voyage of unspeakable beauty.

ANCHORING INTO SELF-TRUST

We've explored in detail how, for the past few thousand years, there has been a campaign to silence, disempower, and control women. To remove us from our intuition and deep feminine knowing. Most women are unaware that this has been happening. Client after client tells me that something has felt "off" for most of their lives, but they had no idea what it was. They tell me they've tried to make sense of a life that always felt like something was missing.

Consider your own experience. Can you remember a time in your life when you had a strong feeling about something? Maybe it was a decision for your career, or about a relationship, or a moment in which you wanted to speak up, or a choice for your child. You sat with that feeling, and it felt like a part of you, but you quickly rationalized away your inner knowing. You told yourself things like "No, that's crazy" or "I should listen to what everyone else is telling me." You tamped down the intuition, and only weeks, months, or years later, you looked back and realized: Your intuition always knew. It was guiding you. Society gaslights us so well that we stop trusting our inner knowing.

So how do you create a more rooted-into-your-soul kind of living in a world that bombards you with the message that you're never enough? Never thin enough, young enough, fertile enough. Never a good enough daughter, wife, mom, religious devotee. Constant patriarchal propaganda leads to self-criticism that pulls away from your ability to feel, and ground into, your deep inner knowing. Pay attention to the ways you doubt yourself, how you seek answers externally rather than internally, how you fail to trust yourself—and how you often betray yourself.

It makes sense why women do these things. We have had constant self-questioning role-modeled by mothers, aunts, and a world culture that raises women to not trust themselves. Notice how lack of self-trust keeps us from accessing our intuition. Because trusting oneself is such a foreign concept, and because many women are disconnected from their inner wisdom, it takes practice and time to learn how to be: to listen, to move, to feel for the answers to our lives.

Self-trust lives within you. To access it, you first must commune with your internal self, the ancient parts of you, the women of centuries ago who knew how to trust intuition and understood that it's our superpower as women. Getting back in touch will require you to feel your way through life, not think your way through. Now, I recognize there are times we must absolutely use our cerebral brains to make decisions, but the vast majority of our lives as women can be run on intuition and divine internal guidance.

LISTEN TO YOUR INTUITION

This ancient intuition and self-trust saved my son's life. When my now twenty-three-year-old son was a toddler, he had dozens of life-threatening food allergies. Our allergy doctor, one of the best in the US, told me there was nothing that could be done. His allergies ruled our entire family life, because even a small bite of one of the more than twenty foods he was allergic to could kill him. I lived every day in fear of another emergency ambulance ride. Of losing my son.

At the time, I was in a support group for parents who had children with severe allergies, and I'd learned about an alternative healer who was using energy, mindset, and oral immunotherapy to cure anaphylaxis. I took down her information, made an appointment, and met with her weeks later.

During that visit, my desperation was traded for hope. Even though her approach was brand-new—one she had designed on her own, and she had few clients and even fewer success stories—my intuition kicked in. As I sat in her office listening to her describe how she could help my son, a feeling washed over me. It was one of knowing, and it flooded my entire body, like I was remembering ancient healing practices.

But as I left her office, my logical brain kicked in. I started downplaying my response, thinking this approach was absolutely absurd. After all, she wasn't even a doctor! She had zero training, and she'd only treated a handful of clients. I left her office thinking I was crazy for even considering it. Six months passed, and every day I thought about whether I should take my son to her and at least try. Then, suddenly, we were moving from Massachusetts to Colorado for my husband's job, so it wasn't an option anymore.

Two years later, endless ambulance rides, and even more food allergies added to the list of what could kill my son, I called the healer to see how I could get my son in to see her. She had a one-year wait list and her only office was in Massachusetts. Her results were 100 percent—every single child had been cured. In my desperation, I begged to be seen sooner, knowing my son might not survive a year. Hearing my need, she asked if I could be there in six weeks, to which I immediately said yes. I was willing to do anything to save my son's life. After a moment, she said, "Amanda, you have to believe. You cannot come here in doubt, or this will not work."

Six weeks later, I packed up our things and moved with my children to Boston for a year; my husband had to stay behind to work. I will never forget the healer's words to me, and I needed that reminder to anchor into my inner wisdom and self-trust, because almost no one else in my life seemed to share my knowing. Every family member, and especially our traditional allergist—the one who had offered no solutions—thought I had lost my mind. "She is not a doctor. What are you thinking?" was the constant refrain.

But they were wrong. My intuition was wise. One year to the date we moved, my son was completely allergy free! And he has remained so, with not a single reaction to any food and no more EpiPens! There was even a book written about our experience and the experiences of other families who sought alternative medicine healings, called *The Other Side of Impossible* by Susannah Meadows.

This was a pivotal experience in my life. My intuition had told me this was the right thing years prior, but I had felt "crazy" for wanting to try and found every excuse to drown out my deep knowing. This journey with my son was the end of doubting my intuition and the beginning of leaning into this mysterious power within me. Almost every choice I now make comes from a deep well within me, and I have released the need to check with others first and make sure they agree. It is an inexplicable liberation that has led to endless beauty in my life.

I share this example as evidence of what's possible when you get underneath your beliefs and assumptions. I invite you to not simply read this book but to immerse yourself into the practice of self-trust. Make this an experiential journey—mine for the gold of your life. Envision this journey to access your ancient wisdom as though you are walking the Camino de Santiago in Spain. Every step is a new discovery; each turn a new vista. A path you have never traveled before. At times, you might feel weary, and at other times, exhilarated. This is a personal pilgrimage, a walk that begins in your soul, a path on which parts of you will be lost and new parts will be found.

As you embark on this journey of rewriting your beliefs, assessing meaning, and building self-trust, you might be enchanted by what feels like a brand-new self-relationship. Allow yourself to be intoxicated by the twists and turns. You're entering a new land for exploring womanhood and an opportunity to deepen into a relationship with yourself like never before. An intimacy with your thoughts, your feelings, your body, your ideologies. Allow yourself to be in wonder. Give yourself the glorious gift of curiosity by asking: Who will I become in this process?

The world I described in the opening of this chapter, the one of communing, nourishment, and replenishment, gets to be yours. But like the healer said to me, you have to believe. And then you have to decide, take action, and be willing to sit with all that you discover along the way. For self-inquiry is the only way you can begin to create a new reality. From there, you must release the systems that have kept you down, which we will explore in the next chapter.

Chapter 4

FREEING YOURSELF FROM SYSTEMS THAT UPHOLD THE DOUBLE STANDARD IN AGING

"I have already settled it for myself so flattery and criticism go down the same drain and I am quite free."

—GEORGIA O'KEEFFE

ON A SUNNY afternoon in 2021, Sarah Jessica Parker and Andy Cohen were spotted out to lunch in Los Angeles. As they enjoyed their meal, they had no idea they were about to go viral.

Soon after, photos of their lunch showed up across the internet, showing them enjoying a meal, each with gray hair. Were the articles and social media posts hinting at a potential collaboration? A new TV show for Parker? Curiosity at their friendship?

No, nope, and definitely not. Instead, the articles dissected Parker's gray hair.

What followed the viral photo were endless slams and nasty criticism about how the gray hair made Sarah Jessica Parker look old. Not Cohen, who had a full head of gray hair in the photo—just Parker. The attacks were cruel and unnecessary, and depicted the exact double standard of aging. The picture eventually prompted online articles in *Today*, *Yahoo!*, *People*, and more.

In a *Vogue* interview later that year, Parker addressed this experience, saying, "There's so much misogynist chatter in response to us that would never. Happen. About. A. Man."[1] In her conviction, she accentuated every word with a clap of her hands.

And Parker is just one example of the pressures and expectations cast on women in the media. Canadian news anchor Lisa LaFlamme, who had worked at CTV News for thirty-five years, was let go after letting her hair go gray during the pandemic. The dismissal started a firestorm globally. With two years left in her contract, and comments from upper management referring to her hair, she was completely devastated to receive news that her long career with the network as a journalist and anchor was over.

In an interview with Katie Couric, LaFlamme points out a particularly important distinction: that when people refer to ageism, they are typically referring to women, not men. Katie Couric goes on to say that, as women age, it is seen as "off-putting and not appealing."[2] She believes this is perpetuated because we have very few, if any, role models of women aging naturally. Women are rewarded by playing the game of never aging and swiftly punished if they do not comply. Often, these terms are unspoken. I'll add that while we're talking about famous women, this pressure applies universally to the female experience. All women are entered in the anti-aging game, whether they know it yet or not.

In previous chapters, we explored the war women are encouraged to wage on our bodies. We've dug into the history of patriarchy, the ways in which we uphold it, and the harm we do to ourselves and our sisters when we hurt ourselves in the name of beauty. But we haven't yet dug deep into the double standard of aging, the punitive systems built to keep us complicit, and the ways society idolizes aging men.

At this point, you might be ready to move on. To get to the solutions. To heal and revolutionize your own womanhood. After all, that's the narrative we hear most of the time: We know patriarchy exists, why dwell on it? Can't we just focus on the solutions?

And we will get to the solutions; we are getting there. But for too long, we have looked past the why, what, and how, and gone straight to fixing. As though if we could just apply the steps one through five of this simple framework—voilà!—problem solved. Now, wasn't that easy? Simple!

But patriarchy is complex, and one of the ways it thrives is through the dichotomy of aging. By the end of this chapter, you'll look at the world around you with new eyes, at the gray-haired men and same-aged women with frozen faces and dyed hair, and want to scream at the screen: Enough!

THE GAME AND THE PUNISHMENT

In May of 2023, I attended a Formula One prerace dinner, where I sat next to a well-known news anchor. Upon learning about my work, she had much to share. She lamented that she was about to turn forty, and was feeling complete terror about the stability of her job. In an effort to secure her status at the network, she was having endless beauty procedures done. A wrinkle or gray hair would send her into a panic, and she was in the never-ending fight to keep them hidden at all costs.

When I inquired about her cohosts, she reported that they were two middle-aged men who had both gone gray and had multiple visible signs of aging. When I invited her to consider how she is perpetuating the storyline of the double standard for women, she adamantly said there was no other option. While we did later go on to discuss her leaving and starting her own show, she felt too overwhelmed by the undertaking and said staying and "playing by the rules" was the easier option.

At the same dinner later that evening, two very influential women, after many glasses of wine and obvious intoxication, approached me.

"Stop pretending to like your gray hair," one of the women said to me. "There is nothing appealing about it."

Her friend, hovering slightly behind her, added, "There's no way your husband really likes it. He's just pretending."

I smiled, meeting their eyes one at a time. "I can see your fear—your fear of aging," I replied. "But to be clear, that fear is yours, not mine."

With the aid of alcohol, these women vocalized what so many women believe. I still wonder if my response sparked something in them, or caused them to sink deeper into their sad beliefs.

Consider why men transition into gray hair with such ease and rarely think about coloring it, while most women are terrified of the thought of letting anyone see their graying roots. What is the message here? That aging is normal for men and catastrophic for women?

As we have been bringing to consciousness all the ways women and men experience aging differently, it's imperative to explore how to divest from, and release, allegiances to the system that holds genders to completely different standards, especially as they age. We must ask the hard questions and then look at the ways in which we perpetuate the storyline.

Questions like: Why, in most parts of the world, are aging men revered while aging women are seen as irrelevant? Why is it that as men age, they are coined "silver fox" or "refined and distinguished," and women are said to have "let themselves go" or are termed "old maid or spinster"? How do we—do I—play a part in this narrative?

We all know that men are celebrated for aging, and that they gain relevance and power as the years pass. And it's perfectly normal to see older men dating younger women, but if the opposite happens, it makes headlines. To know all of this is one thing, but to dig deep into this messaging and undo it within yourself is something entirely different.

And this double standard is physically harming women. I know many women who have had double mastectomies and go on to clean up their eating habits, cut back on alcohol, and add more health routines into their life . . . but when asked about cutting back on facial fillers or stopping hair dye, they look at me like I'm crazy. Like I had just asked the most absurd question possible. They are willing to risk their health, their literal lives, rather than look older. But they will readily admit that a man gets sexier when he ages and laugh off how unfair it is.

It's devastating how deep the brainwashing runs. An Environmental Working Group survey found that, on average, American women put 168 ingredients on their bodies each day, many containing known toxins. The group also found that many of these ingredients were ending up inside people's bodies.[3] Yet it seems women are tone-deaf to this reality, waving this information off as if these ingredients were completely benign. Women are willing to take massive risks for their beauty without really considering the long-term effects of the toxins they are applying, injecting, and consuming.

This duality continues to be perpetuated through lack of representation in the modeling industry. We see aging men grace the billboards and magazines, touted as sexy and refined. Meanwhile, we still see very few mature female models in those same spaces. I know two models who have been in the industry most of their lives. Now, both in their late fifties and still modeling, they deal with endless criticism from men who tell them things like: "Hang it up, Grandma," "We don't want to see you in a bathing suit all wrinkled," and "You look desperate." And it's not just the industry; assaults fly at them every single day on their social media accounts. To make it worse, they've shared with me that their male colleagues receive nothing but support and celebration for their modeling careers.

Beyond modeling, we see the double standard on television. Consider the reality show, *The Golden Bachelor*, which included participants in their sixties and seventies. Like its predecessor, *The Bachelor*, the show features a single man looking for love, with multiple women vying for his affection.

What seemed to offer an opportunity to highlight one's next phase of life instead makes a mockery of aging and feels like yet another million steps away from our divinity as women. The female contestants' obsession with aging permeates the screen as they talk about how happy they are that there are interventions to keep them looking young. The women desperately claw at their youth, willing to do whatever is necessary to look decades younger. The fixation on the external is a devastating crisis. While it's clear that Gerry, the golden bachelor, has made efforts to look good for the show, he also looks like he's in his golden years. The women's ages, on the other hand, appear ambiguous.

Here's the crux of it, from society's point of view: Aging men are safe. Solid. Desirable. Even sexy.

Visibly aging women? Failure. Obsolete. Unworthy of attention or adoration. Need fixing. And definitely not sexy.

See the disconnect here? The dichotomy? The blatant sexism on the screen, in my clients' lives, in my life, in your life too? It's not enough to know we're punished for aging, to understand that patriarchy exists. To fully dismantle patriarchy and revolutionize womanhood, we must uncover the sexist extremes—and call it what it is so we can begin to enact change.

LOSING OUR FACES

As we unpack the difference between how men and women are "allowed" to age, fear becomes a pulsing theme, because punishment is on the table. That a woman dare exist for herself is unthinkable in much of our world. On the most primal level, I believe society fears aging women because they are no longer as easily manipulated. By that logic, men never existed to be manipulated, so society has no reason to be scared of their aging faces.

In a world that infantilizes women, a mature-looking woman represents wisdom and power. She is no longer trying to gain approval or be pleasing. She speaks her truth and knows exactly what she wants. She has a fierceness, a confidence, a knowing that she could not access when she was too busy posing for attention in her younger years. Mature women threaten the very foundation of patriarchy. As a society, we don't know what to do with a woman like that, so we want to make her wrong, make her comply, remember what is expected, get back in the box. How dare she be so free, lest she forget the rules. The audacity of a woman to age in this modern world!

On the contrary, I have always admired the faces of aging women and find them mesmerizing. I adored my grandmother's face with her deep lines, the architecture so captivating, the richness of memories running through each beautiful crevice. When I was in her presence, I studied her with wonder. And when I worked on the Alzheimer's unit as a nurse's aide during my first year of college, one of the things I enjoyed most was washing my patients' faces each night before bed. I was in awe of how much they had seen, lived, and loved. And even though they weren't able to recall their own names, the stories of their lives were etched across their faces.

While society wants us to see aging as a crisis, the real crisis I see is that we are losing the faces of aging women. And what a loss: the art, the landscape, the stories. None of that depth is captured in a frozen face.

The saddest part of this reality is that young girls lack naturally aging role models. Young men, on the other hand, have refined older gentlemen to look to with their gray hair and wisdom lines. Young women crave their own example of another way. This is why, nearly every time I leave my home—whether I am at a local store, in a major metropolitan

> *While society wants us to see aging as a crisis, the real crisis I see is that we are losing the faces of aging women. And what a loss: the art, the landscape, the stories. None of that depth is captured in a frozen face.*

city, or even another country—without fail, young women in their late twenties and early thirties approach me. And in almost every single inter- action, they are in tears.

They tell me a variation of: "Thank you, thank you, thank you for being a voice, a leader for women. We have so few examples—it's really scary. When I fear aging, I come to your page and breathe. My mom is terrified of aging; I have no role model. It's so lonely. All my friends are getting fillers in their faces and tell me to start now as it's preventative." On and on they go, and they never want me to leave, as if they are starving for more inspiration, one more hit of truth. It's overwhelming how desperate and lost these women all seem when it comes to aging. One young woman told me a few weeks ago that she showed her boyfriend my profile and said, "This is how I plan to age: naturally. If you are not OK with that, we may as well break up now."

Can you imagine a man ever needing to say that? To need to have a relationship conversation about his right to age without needles and knives?

Young women deserve better. Think about it: What are we teaching them? To fear aging before they have even entered full adulthood? Placing the majority of one's energy and focus on appearance speaks to our prior- ities. I am deeply saddened for the future and what is being left to young women. Quite honestly, I find it disturbing and psychotic that we are in this place. We have gone so far backward as women. As long as you pose for patriarchy, be very clear, you are not in true agency or power—you are still a pawn in the bigger game. You are still bidding for approval, and there is zero liberation in that.

Consider how much more free time men have for self-actualization, without the hours each week spent on their looks. I often wonder what women would be capable of creating in their lifetime if we put less of our energy into how we look and what needs to be "fixed." What would be possible if we focus on our humanity rather than ourselves as objects for the male gaze? The fixation on looks has taken the form of psychological warfare that seems to be eroding the spirit of women.

Even if not in direct conversation about it, the evidence of this skewed two-pronged storyline of aging is everywhere. The frozen females and deeply creased males; the perceived increasing value of older men and increasing invisibility of older women. As women, the marketing machine and cultural storylines of women needing to look a certain way to be loved, to be chosen, to be worthy, run so profoundly deep that most of us don't realize the psychological grip it has on our lives and the real destruction it causes. The havoc it wreaks on women's overall well-being—health, finances, psyche—is something we have yet to even fully comprehend.

This is where we must examine what we have allowed as women. We must bring into our consciousness the ways in which we continue to give our power away to such a cheap and insulting storyline. The ways we allow men to visibly age with dignity while we treat aging women with disgust. This is where we must question the sum of our lives and the values we want to root into, or we will never gain agency over our aging selves.

THE MUSE MATTERS

Recently, the lack of visible, powerful female aging weighed on me. While I've worked to create a safe space in my platform as The Midlife Muse, I sought additional inspiration, someone who would add fuel to my already flaming mission. For two years, I had looked for someone to anchor to, to draw strength from. I wanted to find a woman grounded in matriarchal, positive aging ideology. A woman who is unshakable. A woman who is aging and not apologizing for it. A woman who is not a performative puppet for the patriarchy.

I was ravenous for a woman who found her own way, her own path, who did not play small or conform to what the world imposed upon her. I wanted to find a woman to learn from who was not controlled by toxic beauty culture and who was certainly not afraid to age. A woman grounded in her truth, not spinning plates of pleasantness.

I searched high and low, but couldn't find her.

For me, this quest was about finding representation in a woman who aged powerfully and with zero apologies. One who was revered and still creating art in her older age. I wanted proof that I could do it too. A muse to inspire me and help me persevere.

So, when my best friend and I took a trip "off grid" to camp in New Mexico for four days a little while back, I knew my mission. The night before we got on the road, we set intentions for the trip and what we hoped to experience. I was highly emotional, and my intention was crystal clear because it had been lodged in my heart for over two years. So as the words flowed out, I was unsurprised at how potent my intention felt in my entire body: to find my muse, a sage, a crone, a woman I could sit at the feet of and learn from.

I never could have imagined what would unfold over the coming days. As we pulled into Ghost Ranch in Abiquiu, New Mexico, I felt magnificence and possibility wash over me; little did I know in that moment that I was entering the land of Georgia O'Keeffe. The vast sky, the red dirt, the enveloping mountains called to my soul in a way that brought me to tears. Moments later, we were standing in the welcome center and waiting to receive information about which campsite we had been assigned for the night. I walked over to an old TV playing a video about the history of Ghost Ranch, took a seat in a dusty metal chair, and listened closely. I was spellbound and speechless as the narrator told the story of Georgia O'Keeffe. I'd heard of O'Keeffe and seen many of her stunning paintings but knew very little about her life. As I watched the film, I knew I needed to learn more about her. Everything about her.

I felt an instantaneous connection to her renegade spirit, her lack of conformity, her freedom, her audacity, her exquisite face etched with deep lines and her gray hair pulled back tightly at the nape of her neck. Her paintings, symbolizing the female body, were boldly edge-pressing for that time. As a budding artist in the 1920s, she overcame every limitation placed on her. When questioned by a deeply religious woman about her late nights out dancing with different men, O'Keeffe responded that it had never occurred to her to not be free.

I found my muse, the woman I had been searching for, in the middle of the desert. I have since studied her life, and I have pictures of her in my office as daily inspiration and reminders of all that matters to me about being a woman who is forging a new path, a way that very few have yet stepped into. Examples matter, and I feel so blessed to have found my muse.

Similarly, you may need to find your muse. Someone to show you that it really is possible to break free from the system of patriarchy, to write your own rules, and to age unapologetically.

So where can you start? You can look around you, like I did, trying to find the right-fit woman to inspire you. It could be an artist or celebrity or your grandmother. But if you find, like me, that those examples are hard or impossible to find, you can also immerse yourself in community. A place to begin could be joining an online group or a local meetup, or hosting your own event, like I did all those years ago. When you connect with women who are on this similar journey, you open yourself up to being a muse for others, and also meeting the women who will become your muses.

As a clinical psychologist, I know that muses matter, so much so that I started an online community membership, The Muses. Examples and leadership help us to overcome feelings of confusion and shame. One cannot simultaneously feel shame for aging and hold profound self-love. Shame is pervasive and erodes the human soul. I watch it daily: women running around claiming happiness and spirituality, while inwardly hating themselves.

But once women find their muse and community, everything changes. They're exposed to other ways of thinking about what it means to be a woman and new philosophies rooted in matriarchy, body honor, and the spirituality of aging. After all, there is nothing more spiritual than watching yourself age as a woman in this modern world.

FINDING THE SPIRITUALITY OF AGING WITH THE MIRROR PRACTICE

When women ask me about my spiritual practices—crystals? oracle cards? journaling?—I assure them that my number one spiritual practice is watching myself age, not fighting it, not apologizing for it or covering it up. It's walking through the world with my shoulders back and head held high; my voice that speaks without apology; my silver hair and wrinkles not simply on display but carried with profound reverence.

By choosing to see aging as a spiritual experience, I remain curious about who I become on this journey. And I deeply understand that I must merge with the process rather than shame it or bypass it.

We miss the journey, the magic of our lives, when we do not surrender to natural processes. You can choose to see aging as a spiritual experience too—like my client, who sat down with her husband and told him she was stopping Botox and felt excited about her changing face. Or like my other client, who told her partner that she would be aging naturally, and if he had a problem with it, they didn't have a future together. These women chose to see themselves age, fully and naturally, and invited the men in their lives to journey with them . . . or opt out. Only they could make a choice to own their spiritual journeys; only you can make a choice to own yours.

When I stopped coloring my hair several years ago, many women asked if I planned to have a stylist professionally transition me to silver so I wouldn't have to go through the "awkward" phases of growing it out. I was shocked at the continual question but even more so by their dismay when I responded that I was excited to see who I would become along the way. I am saddened at how few women have ever even considered that there could be something so profound, so potent, to be gained along the path of aging.

As the leading consumers in the world, women hold limitless power to change the storyline, but that can't begin to happen until they see themselves differently—until they recognize their value and worth. I hope this book serves as a reminder of your inherent power and divinity. That worthiness will never come from outside of you but only from the inner work you are willing to do. Self-love creates an unshakable foundation. Unless you are willing to acknowledge and feel the fury of the brainwashing you have been subject to, you'll continue to downplay the effects of chasing external validation and the ways it is ruining your life, creating anxiety and desperation for approval. Your liberation is in your hands alone, and you must be willing to free yourself from the cage and write a different way forward.

And the new way forward is this: embracing the idea of aging as a profound spiritual journey and experiencing all of the lessons and power along the way. You cannot simultaneously try to cover up your aging, rail against it, *and* feel into the spirituality of it. Instead, I encourage you to breathe, to see the magic, to divest from messaging that is "anti" aging and to practice aging in a way that feels nourishing, true, ancient, and holy to your nervous system. To no longer equate aging with being damaged.

This work requires radical responsibility and self-leadership. It requires being in love with yourself. In awe.

My greatest teacher in self-love was my baby. I had just taken my nine-month-old daughter out of the bath—this was twenty years ago—and while I was cleaning up, I noticed she had crawled over to a huge mirror and pulled herself up to a standing position in front of it. As she interacted with her reflection, I noticed that she was experiencing pure awe and wonder. I reached for my camera to take a photo and capture the precious moment forever. Little did I realize the impact that moment would have many years later, on thousands of women.

Just a few years ago, I was sorting through old photos when I stumbled across this adorable picture. I became transfixed by every detail of her face: captivated by the way she looked into her own eyes in the mirror, overwhelmed with the innocence of it all. And I also wondered, "When do girls stop looking at themselves like this?" As I tucked the photo away, I felt a stirring, for what exactly I was not certain of at the moment. I just knew

I wanted to incorporate an element of this decades-ago moment into my work with women.

I decided to start with myself, as I do with any practice before I bring it to my clients and community. Soon after, I began a ninety-day mirror practice. Every morning when I woke, I would make my way to the mirror. No checking my phone or allowing the outside world to contaminate the tenderness of my sleepy self. I committed to standing at the mirror for approximately three minutes. I started with ninety seconds and extended the time as I became more accustomed to the practice. My intention was to only look through the eyes of curiosity, with zero judgment or focusing on "flaws" or how tired I looked. Only love. Only humanity. Only divinity. I allowed eye contact with myself, and deep presence with my being, to be the energy that led the practice. I was absolutely astounded by what transpired over the three months.

The first several days were awkward. Time seemed to drag on and all I could see were my tired eyes, my sunspots, my aging skin. I initially felt a deep sadness, not for the way I looked but for the pressure I felt deep inside to even focus on how I looked over how I felt. Eventually, I decided I could stand there and be in neutrality. I didn't have to rush to feel anything profound or to force wonder. Allowing the process to unfold naturally was the best way I found to approach the mirror practice.

There is history attached to our female faces and what we see in our reflections. What I discovered through this process was so profound I wanted to incorporate it into my work in the world. I understood that without this fundamental seeing of our own souls, nothing would ever actually change. This practice, when done regularly, taps into something at the deep nervous-system level. It was as if I saw deeper layers of myself each day I stood there. Over time, I began to feel profound gratitude for all the times my body has shown up for me, deep compassion for all the ways I kept going when I felt defeated, and unspeakable love for myself and my humanity. But this took time. I was not able to access self-awe as easily before I started the mirror practice. The holiness of the practice started to change me on a cellular level. I reset the way I approach seeing and experiencing myself in the world. I'm no longer primed for the way the world conditions women, through the lens of lack and what needs to be fixed. Today I honor my soul.

I now teach this practice at my retreats, and it is always a profound experience for women as they take their place at the mirror and truly see themselves. Most of the women cry at the realization of how few times, if ever, they have come to the mirror through the eyes of reverence.

I encourage you to give yourself this beautiful gift of the mirror practice. Allow yourself to see every moment as unwrapping the most exquisite gift, the gift of your life, right before your very eyes. Fundamentally changing the way you love yourself requires embracing a new mindset, new practices, new rituals, and new beliefs. You must divest from toxic beauty culture, and connect into self-reverence, if you ever want to have a healthy, loving relationship with your body and the process of aging.

Chapter 5

FROM SELF-LOATHING
TO SELF-HONOR

"Nobody can make you feel inferior without your consent."
—ELEANOR ROOSEVELT

IN 2014, THE menstruation brand Always released a commercial called "Run Like a Girl." The video launched the start of their incredible campaign, #LikeAGirl, which tackled the societal harm on a young girl's confidence during puberty. The video begins by asking adolescents and young adults—mostly female—to "run like a girl." Each participant is brought in individually so as not to influence their answers. Standing before a dark blue-gray backdrop, they respond to the question by jogging in place with their arms flailing about, with one participant joking, "My hair!" They're then asked to throw like a girl, which elicits a lot of weak grunting, T-rex-arms, and pretend-dropping an invisible ball.

The message: Girls can't run or throw.

Then they bring in girls ages ten and younger. They are asked the same question, but this time the participants respond by running and throwing with all their might. One girl sprints from end to end in the room, another runs in place as fast as she can, and yet another demonstrates a powerful baseball pitch. On the screen, the ad reads, "A girl's confidence plummets during puberty."

The producers then ask the older females to share their reflections on how the term "run like a girl" has impacted them as they've grown, noting that it's usually between the ages of ten and twelve that they first hear this used as an insult. The girls reflect on the harmful messaging that they aren't seen as being as capable as boys, and how that messaging negatively impacted them as they grew. They are given the opportunity to redo their running and throwing, and they move powerfully and confidently. The commercial ends with a young woman asking: "Why can't 'run like a girl' also mean win the race?"[1]

This powerful three-minute commercial illustrates the immense power that social conditioning plays in our lives and the influence of these negative messages as we grow. And of course, it's not just you and me experiencing it—it's also your mother, sister, daughter, female friends, and every other woman and girl you care about. If you haven't seen the ad yet, I highly recommend doing a quick online search and watching it yourself.

While the campaign is more than a decade old, current data confirms this disturbing story about coming of age as a girl in the United States. Studies show that up to 60 percent of elementary school girls worry about their weight. They start dieting around the same age too, with girls as young as nine reporting that they're on weight-loss diets "very often." And by the tender age of thirteen, more than half of girls—53 percent—say they are "unhappy with their bodies." By seventeen, that number skyrockets to 73 percent.[2]

Take a moment to visualize this. Imagine a room of one hundred young girls. Fifty-three of them are dressed head to toe in black, representing negative self-thoughts; forty-seven are in sunshine yellow, representing positive self-image. Twenty of the vibrant, life-filled girls exit, and when they come back, they are sullen and dressed in all black. Now, seventy-three girls stand in black, their bodies slumped, a representation of their inner thoughts. Only twenty-seven sunny, smiling girls remain. Worse yet, statistics show that 45.5 percent of the girls in our illustrative room have already thought about getting cosmetic surgery.[3]

This is unacceptable. And as they get older, the self-loathing often turns to physical self-harm. As we've discussed, women eventually have access to cosmetic surgery, beauty products containing toxins, and endless opportunities on social media for further annihilation of their confidence.

We've explored how women are born into the lie that their worth needs to be earned—to be granted by anyone other than themselves. And we've discussed how, between the ages of six and twelve years old, the average girl begins the most devasting internal battle, one that will go on for her entire lifetime and pervade the majority of her experiences. Her need to be externally validated will contaminate the way she perceives herself and all other women. At best, she will be self-conscious and self-critical; at worst, she will self-loathe and self-terrorize. Either state is a disease that ravishes her mind, body, and spirit and robs her of actualizing self-love. As she ages, the anti-female machine only grows louder and more destructive as so many women are afraid to turn the battle outward and recognize the real enemy: a culture that sells women on the belief they need to be smaller, quieter, and more pleasing.

But it's not her—not *your*—fault. It *is* your responsibility to claim self-love and reconnect to the parts of yourself that you've abandoned.

In this chapter, we will explore how to become a beautiful vessel of self-love and self-reverence, carry a deep sense of inner beauty, and embody profound worthiness rooted in the belief of being a sacred, divine being. I have seen countless clients build a remarkable life that they never before imagined possible. If you're willing, you can have anything you want—and surpass even your wildest dreams.

RECREATE THE IMPRINT

More than likely, you are not eight years old right now. So, if you're reading this at twenty-four, fifty-two, or seventy-one, isn't the damage already done? You can't go back and undo the past . . . right?

That's true. But while you can't change what has happened to you, you can reconnect to the child within, your young self who experienced the hurt, who began a journey of self-lack from such a young age. And from that place of awareness, you can recreate the imprint that moment made on your life.

We women are often disconnected to earlier versions of ourselves. We tuck the memories away and hope we can move on from them. The truth is, our early experiences create an imprint and often deeply impact how we interact with the world, the way we feel about our bodies, and even our entire female existence. Achieving true self-love requires connecting to your younger self and understanding your early experiences of being in a female body.

Like all of my clients, I bet there was a disconnection point for you. A moment or series of experiences that severed your confidence. Sometimes it is a major trauma; other times, it is a shaming conversation with a loved one.

When I ask my clients to recount the first time they heard a comment, insult, or suggestion about their bodies, most of them remember a moment between the ages of eight and ten. When prompted, they are able to recall in great detail what was said, who said it, and the feelings of shame that washed over them. They remember that first cut, first insult, and first realization that others had expectations of them and how they should be in the world.

One such example is a client we'll call Greta. This client spent the majority of her life at war with her body and carried immense shame about her weight; to understand the root of this shame, I helped her unlock an early childhood memory. During a guided meditation, she was able to access an experience from when she was ten years old. It was a memory so painful she had been unconscious of it until that moment, when she made the conscious choice to access it—almost as though her brain had tucked it away in a "no access" zone to protect her.

In vivid detail, Greta recalled it being Easter morning. She was getting ready to go to church. Little Greta was so excited to put on the new dress that her mom had bought for her months earlier. As she walked into the kitchen, proud as ever and feeling like a princess, she was expecting her parents to ooh and aah over her beauty; instead, they had the opposite reaction.

Her father did not hide his disapproval and outright disgust. He told her she looked ridiculous in the dress because it was too tight and made for a girl who was not so fat. Her mom went on to explain that she had no idea what happened, because when they'd bought the dress a few months earlier, it fit perfectly.

"She's obviously grown since then," her mother stated.

"Grown?" her father replied, his tone angry. "She is huge. She's exploding out of the dress. She looks ridiculous in it." He then demanded she take it off and put on something that fit her.

Through tears and hot shame, Greta ran back to her room. All she wanted to do was hide. She loved the dress, she had felt fancy and beautiful before she showed her parents, but now all she felt was embarrassed for existing. She searched her drawers and closet for something else to wear and, in that moment, began her lifelong journey of profound shame for her body, hiding it behind extra-large clothes and forever apologizing for taking up any space. To this day, her father still makes comments about her body when she comes home to visit, each time further reinforcing her feelings of self-loathing.

Greta's first step to undoing shame and accessing self-love was remembering this moment. She had to feel it fully, love that little girl version of herself, and understand how her relationship with her father was contributing to her shame cycle. That meditation was the start of her self-love journey.

In my work with women, I take them on a variety of journeys deep into themselves. One of those magical journeys is into an uncharted territory we rarely speak of, an area of mystery that also carries taboo: the womb. It is a place of creation, limitless potential, and often where endless pain and trauma are stored. I set the context for the importance of meeting, and connecting with, their inner maiden, their younger self, the one who often felt slighted, shamed, forgotten, and rejected.

Now, I'll ask you: When was the first time you heard a comment, insult, or suggestion about your body that made you feel ashamed? Take some time now to connect to that experience. Close your eyes, breathe deep, and scan your memories.

> *When was the first time you heard a comment, insult, or suggestion about your body that made you feel ashamed?*

Identifying this moment allows you to understand when, where, and how loss of self-love began. Context matters in your healing journey. On the other hand, remaining unconscious to these moments keeps you disconnected from yourself. Healing feels more elusive when you cannot connect your past to your present.

Now imagine taking that young version of you, scooping her up and placing her onto your lap. What do you want to say to her? What words do you wish she had heard as a little girl? Can you assure her that she never should have been spoken to that way? That those words she heard were projections of someone else's fear? Can you promise her that she is now safe with you, that she will be respected and honored every single day?

Often, our parents or caregivers were not able to provide a foundation for self-love, and the damage is best repaired when we learn how to parent ourselves. You start to reparent yourself by speaking words of love and showing up with compassion and patience for yourself now. This is the road to true healing and rewriting a new narrative for your life.

CONNECTING WITH YOUR INNER MAIDEN

Like Greta, we each have a first shame moment—and many more after that initial one. And from this shame begins a lifetime of struggling to love ourselves, especially when it has not been modeled for us. But like a wound, this shame can be healed. Now that you've uncovered your earliest feeling of shame, the next step toward healing is to connect to your younger self and help her re-experience that moment through a lens of self-love.

Let's begin now. Allow yourself uninterrupted time for this inward journey. First, create a beautifully sacred space for yourself. Light some candles and make sure you are dressed in clothing that feels comfortable and flowy, with nothing restricting your womb space. The aim is to create a sense of openness and invitation in both your environment and attire.

Start by taking a few deep, slow breaths. Fill up your chest, lungs, and all the way down into your womb and the space surrounding it. Doing so activates your connection to the area of your body that holds the majority of your pain, trauma, and memories. Your womb space is also the portal of endless creation and holds the frequency of limitless potential. It's important to note this is also the part of a woman's body that carries endless cultural and religious shame, profound responsibility, and fear. We'll circle back to explore these complex relationships even further.

I invite you to close your eyes and craft a mental picture of the inside of your womb. As you gently descend, what do you feel? What do you see? Is it dark, safe, and warm? Does it feel like a place to seek shelter and solace, or does it feel like forbidden territory, unknown and uninviting? As you imagine moving around and exploring inside your womb, notice what energy you feel. Do you feel uncertain, at ease, fearful, exhilarated, or something else entirely?

Now, take a moment and invite your inner maiden, your little girl self, to join you. Maybe she is already there: stuck, scared, angry, sad, and forgotten. Possibly she has been there hiding for many years, afraid to fully emerge. Take a few moments to really see her. Be patient and use your senses to look, listen, and feel her energy. How does your inner maiden present? What does she want to communicate? She may be curious as to where you have been and why it has taken you so long to visit her. She may be mistrustful because she has felt abandoned and all alone. Maybe she feels stifled because you haven't allowed her to express her individuality. Conforming for so long has worn her down. Or maybe she is playful and whimsical and thrilled to see you.

Regardless of how she shows up, this is an opportunity to reassure your little one that you will never hide her away again; you will never silence her or feel ashamed of her. This is a pivotal moment to create a new way of being and relating to yourself—and to reclaim the younger, more vulnerable versions of you. Reconnecting to your inner maiden will be incredibly important as you continue to journey through this book— you're doing this work not only for who you are now but also all the previous versions of you that need healing. This is a beautiful practice to return to, as it will help you connect with different versions of you: your five-year-old self, your twelve-year-old self, your teenage self. You likely experienced many shame moments during girlhood, the kind of shame that silenced the younger you, made you pull inward, and caused you to lose your voice. Each womb meditation is an opportunity to connect with, understand, and begin to heal the damage done to the many younger versions of yourself.

Early life experiences make a profound impact on how and who you are in the world. Bringing them into consciousness allows your life to make more sense. When you are conscious of the impact of shame moments, you have a better chance of fully understanding yourself and create the opportunity for real healing. After all, you can't heal that which you are not conscious of.

The alternative? A lifetime with hidden, unhealed wounds. And sister, that life isn't for you. You've come too far to turn your back on your inner maiden now.

Of course, it's one thing to be in a safe space with lit candles, flowy clothing, and a sense of deep inner connection. What about when you—and your inner maiden—venture out into the world? What about when you open Instagram or get together with relatives or chat with the other moms at drop-off? What about the violence and misogyny and toxic patriarchy we inevitably swim in on a daily basis?

As we've explored in depth, the female body is critiqued, fracked, objectified, profiteered, shamed, and celebrated. The majority of consumerism revolves around how a woman looks, what she can do to look better, smaller, prettier, younger . . . the never-ending list of expectations goes on and on. Ten years ago, as I really began to explore the war women were having with their own bodies, I realized I'd never had a single client, friend, or family member who was not fighting an internal battle with her body. The conditioning runs layers deep, and most women share with me that they have never known internal peace. From a young age, they've been hyper-aware of what needs to be "fixed" and felt shame at not meeting society's physical ideal.

How, then, are we as women ever to overcome this constant internal battle? Bringing this to you, let me ask: Now that you've connected to your inner maiden, how do you become a matriarchal revolutionary? How do you change your internal narrative when negative messages are constantly barraging you, and when every one of your female friends are also struggling? How do you construct a new way forward when the brainwashing machine has been running incognito for your entire lifetime, powerfully and secretly impacting your thoughts and actions?

The path to self-love requires flipping the script. You must take a hard look at the patriarchy and decide to move from feeling ashamed to feeling insulted. We didn't light the patriarchal fire, but it's absolutely our responsibility to snuff it out and light a new fire of self-love. And that flame within, when joined with others, can change the world.

To become a walking revolutionary, to exist in the energy of self-love and to engage in the spiritual experience of being in a human body, you will need to change the beliefs you carry and the messaging you operate from. It is difficult to create a beautiful experience of being human from a toxic foundation of beliefs. We addressed beliefs earlier in the book. Now, with a connection to your inner maiden, you can do even deeper work in this area.

This is where that flipped script comes in. Stepping fully into this work—and into an entirely new way of living—requires fury. It demands outrage. In my own journey, I recognized that creating a new relationship with my body necessitated massive amounts of curiosity and a willingness to truly unpack where I was operating from, *and* I also had to feel rage at all the destructive messaging I had absorbed. This same approach has helped my clients recreate their internal beliefs and love themselves again.

You can begin to flip the script by shifting the time and energy you spend berating and contorting yourself and instead use those resources to challenge and reconstruct the narrative. Consider the hours spent on maintenance appointments, not to mention daily upkeep: applying makeup, doing hair, dressing just so. Imagine what would be possible if all women reclaimed those hours! Envision what we could create with that amount of time, energy, and money—by using our resources to change the world rather than our bodies. The positive impact would span generations.

Redirecting your resources is an act of revolutionary self-love and reclamation. Decide here and now that only you are responsible for how you feel about yourself, about what messaging you will allow to lead your life. In this beautiful moment, dedicate your life to self-honor.

CHANGE YOUR BELIEFS BY ASKING QUESTIONS

As we've explored, shifting how you think and operate requires changing your beliefs about almost everything. If this feels overwhelming, I suggest recasting this next stage of life as an opportunity to finally open the door of a cage you have been stuck inside your entire life. You've been cramped in a small space and have had to contort your body to find comfort. But that comfort never comes. Right now is your moment to begin the walk of liberation and a self-defined lifestyle, one in which radical responsibility is welcomed with pride and excitement.

Now is when you can begin the internal questioning, the exploration of everything you once believed. It's essential to ask endless questions and to be curious about every belief you hold. Questions like:

- Where did I learn that women lose their value as they age?
- Do I fundamentally believe that a woman becomes less worthy as she grows older, or is that a conditioned way of thinking—one that devalues and dehumanizes?
- Is it possible my view of aging comes from a colonized lens of the world?
- Is it possible my beliefs are a byproduct of patriarchy infantilizing women and women falling for the trap of eternal youth as their only value?

Becoming a revolutionary woman requires examining every toxic belief you hold. You need to understand why the belief exists, what role it plays in society, and how it serves men. And you must recognize the absolute power that patriarchy has played in the formation of your life and choices as a woman. As you do, you'll see the ways you have been under a spell, often making decisions without even questioning why.

I equate this journey of awareness to being a young child and listening to your caregivers; you were likely on autopilot, never pausing to question their rules, truths, or expectations. You moved through childhood believing your caregivers knew absolutely everything and that all families thought and operated like yours. It is an innocent, naïve approach but perfectly age-appropriate for a young child. It wasn't until you got older, left your family home and experienced the world—including other perspectives and ways of life—that you realized there are many other approaches to life and family. The range of beliefs are endless! As you explored the world, your mind began to open, and you began questioning everything you once believed. You took the journey of discovering who you are, and what values and beliefs you want to identify with, and you built a life from these pillars.

Unfortunately, you weren't building these beliefs without external influence. As we've seen, patriarchy has infiltrated everything, everywhere, in the world. It has overtaken all systems—religious, medical, workforce, marriage, leadership, entertainment, and beyond to the extent that it is almost impossible to realize you are inside its influence, its sickness. In the same way a fish doesn't know it's swimming in water, most women have no conscious connection to the fact every aspect of their life is informed by being raised within the patriarchal structure. This work of rewriting your beliefs will require you to be fierce, steadfast, relentless, and passionate about identifying, excavating, and healing from a profoundly ill system that has had powerful control over your entire life.

This may be the point where you want to slam this book down, bury your head in the sand, and resign yourself to defeat. You might want to tell yourself it's too much work or, worse yet, delude yourself into believing it's "not really that big of a deal." I want to lovingly remind you that, no matter which direction you go or what you choose, you will never be free until you do this work and disentangle yourself from the ways patriarchy has contaminated your life. And I also want to encourage you with the fact that you've already done some of the work, just by making it this far in the book. Just by reading, you've confronted things most women will never question. You've chosen to keep going. You've opened yourself up to the possibility of a more beautiful future. That takes courage—and you can keep choosing the brave path forward.

The women who opt out of awareness stay in shitty relationships. They remain under the patriarchal spell, believing it's their job to put up with poor behavior from men—that having a breadcrumb relationship is better than being alone. That they are needy and unrealistic if they desire a feast from their relationship. Women who choose to not do this work settle for low pay, are unable to set healthy boundaries, are at war with their bodies for life, believe their only value and power is in how youthful they look, are threatened by and in competition with other women, use loads of toxic beauty products that cause cancer and autoimmune diseases, perform for the male gaze, and use endless numbing mechanisms like drinking, prescription pills, shopping, endless scrolling, and binge-eating to cope with the never-ending ache.

On the other hand, doing the work requires a conviction that pulses through your veins. This work is not for the faint of heart, but I believe every single woman has the power to free herself. Every woman has the opportunity to liberate herself from the invisible shackles she has been bound in since birth and join a sisterhood that is quaking with rage and seeking liberation.

CONSCIOUSLY EXCAVATE THE TRUTH

You started rewriting your beliefs in chapter three, when you made a list of what it means to be a woman. Continuing your belief-rewriting journey involves observing yourself: your thoughts, the messages you tell yourself, the behaviors you engage in, and the belief systems you hold allegiance to. Rather than moving through your life unconsciously, you must be in conscious observation and curiosity about why you feel the way you do. This awareness is the ticket to deeply understanding yourself. This is how you build intimacy with yourself.

It is from this powerful place of self-understanding that you'll begin to regain control from a system that is profiting off of your insecurities.

To begin this quest into what feels most true for you, start paying attention to how you feel most of the time. What thoughts pervade your mind? When I ask my clients this question, they typically report feeling consumed by thoughts of not being pretty enough, thin enough, young enough, and good enough, and they spend a great deal of their free time searching for "enough" in yet another product. Once you develop awareness, the next step is to question those thoughts.

Because we as women have not been raised to go inward and question our thoughts, feelings, and decisions, we rely on quick fixes: "Oh, you don't feel great? Take a pill." "You're feeling unattractive? Buy these potions." This vicious cycle only ends when we take radical responsibility to sit with, observe, and question *why* we are making the decisions we are making.

Doing this will require you to be wildly brave, even courageous enough to be the outlier in a world where most are not asking these hard questions. Because true aliveness, radiance, health, and joy are not found in being unconscious, numb, and controlled. You can liberate yourself from the inside out and be fully free! But first, you must understand the underlying operating system of your consciousness. Otherwise, you'll have nothing more than cheap, quick fixes that don't work and don't last.

My work excavates from the roots of the disease. To do a personal excavation for the truth can be incredibly uncomfortable because it will bring painful points of awareness to the surface, and it is impossible to unsee what has been revealed. I believe this truth-facing is one of the main reasons many women avoid any kind of deep personal development. After all, it's easier to exist on the surface of their lives, never questioning anything and believing they would not have the strength to make the changes required. I get the resistance. In my own life, becoming fully conscious and aware of the ways in which I was complicit in the patriarchy has been difficult to see and admit.

For example, I noticed my own complicity at parties, when someone made a sexist joke and I said nothing. Sometimes I would even laugh a bit. I cringed when I realized I had assumed a doctor a friend was speaking about was a man. I recognized that I kept friendships because others expected me to, not because they were nourishing to my soul. With this awareness, I spent years disentangling myself, my beliefs, my life, and my relationships—and it was exhausting. There were even brief moments when I thought it would have just been better to stay unaware.

Ultimately, doing this work illuminates all of the invisible operating systems by which you live your life. You're choosing to excavate suffering, to lay it bare, and to finally face the ways in which you're participating in your own pain. And make no mistake: The majority of the women I speak with are suffering—and they're doing so silently. They're unhappy in their relationships, disassociated from their bodies, judging themselves for their huge range of emotions, or being told they are unstable and consequently medicated—or all of the above. Each woman I've met has shared a story of numbness, dissatisfaction, or longing, and the most heartbreaking thing is most of them have tried everything they could think of to get relief, and with each attempt came up empty.

IT'S NOT YOU, IT'S THE CULTURE

Women I work with have often been in traditional therapy for fifteen to twenty years, and after just two months of working with me, they report feeling so much better. Many of my clients had been on antidepressants for two decades, and after finally understanding the root of their suffering, and how to honor themselves, their bodies, and their intuition, they no longer wanted to be disconnected from their source. Once women understand that there is nothing "wrong" with them, everything changes. When they finally comprehend that there is *everything* wrong with a culture and system that wants to keep women small, quiet, pleasing, and in service, they also recognize that the actual disease is existing within a system that doesn't allow their full expression.

Coming alive to your life is the absolute greatest gift and healing elixir available. These systems profit from you never feeling enough, so it is important to deeply understand that the only way to true fulfillment is through sourcing your sense of "enough" from within. This is the game-changing moment that I get to witness with my clients: when they connect to the truth that they never needed to be approved of by anyone. From this awareness, they then begin to reconstruct their life. It's like they're coming alive for the first time.

Remember young Greta feeling fancy in her Easter dress? The deep shame she carried around ruled her life. Everything changed for her once she uncovered the fact that the source of her shame was that Easter morning, realized that the only approval she needed was her own, and did the work to rewrite her beliefs. She finally understood that her father's fear was not hers. He was the one who believed women must look a certain way to be valuable, loved, and successful. Greta realized this belief didn't feel aligned for her, and she decided to no longer allow him to speak to her in such a judgmental and critical way.

She became so anchored in self-love that, on a recent visit to see her father, he commented on her weight. She looked directly at him and said, "Let me be very clear about something. Comments about my body or my physical appearance, in any way, are no longer allowed. If you want me in your life, you are going to have to find new ways to engage with me."

This is the power of doing the work of understanding where the shame started, examining if it is a belief that aligns for you, and then setting boundaries around how others are allowed to treat you.

Just as there was more to Greta's story, there can be more to yours too. The process begins with a heart of curiosity and a willingness to explore your own humanity, including your choices. The most loving way to do this is with a foundation of self-love. When you think about all the women in your life—your mother, grandmothers, aunts, mentors, close friends, colleagues—are you able to identify any that were grounded in self-love, the kind of steady-like-an-oak-tree rootedness? Can you name a woman so filled up by her own soulfulness and self-approval that it was magical to witness? Most women I ask can't name one woman who embodies self-love.

Most women have never been raised by, or had proximity to, a woman who was overflowing with self-love. It is an elusive concept, one that feels more like a phrase splashed across a journal than a true embodiment.

As a generational changemaker, you get to be one of the first in your lineage to build a foundation of self-love. We are doing some of that work here. If you want to deepen your journey, one place to continue this work is my self-love online course, which walks you through generational healing: forgiveness, understanding, and awareness of your conditioning, as well as the releasing and rewriting of fundamental beliefs.

The journey to self-love is one of devotion and practice. As women, we have not been coded to love ourselves. Quite the opposite. All we need to do is look at the endless messaging that steals from a woman's sense of internal love. Often, women are even warned to not become "too full of themselves."

In my work with women, self-love is a lifestyle and the base of everything we source from, because without building there first, the foundation is unstable. Developing self-love takes a daily practice of sourcing from within—for your truth and for the messaging on which you want to build a life. Let's look at one practice to help you begin building this foundation.

YOUR EXQUISITE LIFE

Self-love leads to an exquisite life—one that is fueled from a deep sense of inner beauty, not ever-changing trends. It nurtures a phenomenal life steeped in unshakable self-worth, not decisions by others. It supports a sensational life rooted in the belief that you are a sacred, divine being, not an object for pleasing others. Self-love, in essence, is the foundation of a devotional life: an entire way of being that fully supports these qualities of living. Without profound intention, the world's loud messaging will carry you away in its ever-moving current and drown any chance of mastering self-love.

Let me share how I have developed a devotional life and what I recommend to my clients who want to build a solid foundation of self-love. I avoid any and all social media accounts that are toxic in messaging, I choose not to watch any reality television, and watch only those movies that have a soulful, nourishing tone. I do not hang out with people who primarily talk about other people or things, as I prefer ideas. I surround myself with people who are not victims, who seek growth, love, and harmony for all people and the planet. I do not punish my body with tight clothing. I do not apply toxins onto my skin, nor do I inject them in an attempt to look younger. I keep my mindset clean with the most exquisite, kind, loving messages to myself. I honor my body by resting, laughing, playing, dancing, orgasming, consuming healthy foods and beverages, and by starting each day in the mirror honoring my humanity. I am a temple and I treat myself accordingly. I do not allow cheap messaging from a sick world to contaminate me. As the Queen of my life, it is my responsibility to curate the life I dream of, the love I want to feel, and the magic I want to make. I wait for no one. I lead myself. I love myself.

This is my suggestion to you, sister. After all, no one is coming to save you.

As you engage in your own devotional practices, pay attention to all the external factors that will try to take your power away. That will want you to return to your inner battlefield. Notice how others react when you set new boundaries and create new standards for your up-leveled life. Many will feel betrayed, let down, and left behind. Some will feel threatened, triggered, and pissed off. Others will feel that you are asking too much, being unrealistic, or have lost your damn mind. There will even be lovers, partners, dear friends, and family who will try to pull you back into your original ways of being, the way you were when they met you. Often, this is an attempt to keep you in their life, because they fear your growth and are unwilling to grow with you. You will have to decide who you would rather betray: yourself or their low standards.

As we've explored, the world prefers women who are timid, voiceless, and amenable, so when you come out of your decades-long slumber and awaken into full consciousness, it will ignite the majority to call you high maintenance, inconvenient, and a crazy bitch. Be careful of this gaslighting technique meant to quiet you, because it is pervasive in the patriarchy. I encourage you to let others' judgments and fears be theirs. Anchor into *you*.

As you develop a foundation of self-love, the next step is to move fully into your Queendom. And let's be clear: The journey is no fairy tale. But it will provide the happiest ever after of all.

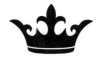

Section III

REWRITING
THE STORY

Chapter 6

FROM PRINCESS
TO QUEEN

"Think like a queen. A queen is not afraid to fail.
Failure is another stepping stone to greatness."

—OPRAH WINFREY

FAIRY TALES WERE an early imprint that taught me so much about being a woman. The lesson: As long as I was pretty, quiet, and helpless, I would be rescued by a prince. In his arms and by his side, my life would finally be worthy. He would save me from the dangers of the world, especially the misery caused by the evil stepmother—another early lesson, that women couldn't be trusted and would always try to silence you.

Consider Sleeping Beauty, who was sentenced to death by the wicked Maleficent at the age of sixteen because of the witch's jealousy. Or Snow White, whose own stepmother ordered the young girl's murder because she was envious of Snow White's beauty, and when the hit failed, tried to poison her with an apple. Or Cinderella, who was essentially enslaved by her stepmother and stepsisters, all of whom were jealous of her beauty. Or Rapunzel, who was stolen as a child and imprisoned in a tower so the evil witch could remain eternally youthful.

Need I go on?

While it's true we also see the trope of the fairy godmother in some of these films, her presence is limited and fleeting, and only there to counteract the evil older woman who is so overcome with feelings of rage over another's beauty, she is willing to kidnap, abuse, and kill.

My worldview didn't change much when I became a teenager, and fairy tales were replaced with romantic comedies. Instead of princesses, I watched movies with the same basic plot featuring a desperate woman willing to settle for cheap love at any cost. These stories further perpetuated the myth of a woman's main role in life: to find love. For without it, she was doomed.

Early indoctrination has created a world of women who seek rather than become. Women who ache for outside validation and approval rather than anchor in their own self-approval. The programming runs so deep that most women are not even conscious of their internal operating systems. Most have never even questioned the rules of engagement.

Where is the nuance and depth in the women on the screen? Why do female characters have little to offer but their youth and beauty? Why do women around the world center men in every aspect of their lives? And why do they receive the message that to do otherwise is a selfish and unworthy pursuit?

The answer to these questions isn't hard to find: Female characters are almost exclusively written by men. Earlier, we explored how men make up 91 percent of fictional film directors—and that number extends beyond the director's seat, to the writers. Even by 2021, the World Economic Forum reported that men make up 83 percent of movie directors and writers.[1] Let's pause on that number for a moment. In a room of one hundred directors and writers, there would be only seventeen women—a staggeringly low percentage of women influencing what happens on screen. This statistic is just one of many equity issues in filmmaking.

No wonder we are fed such a limited perspective and simple, love-starved female characters! We're raised on storytelling from a man's perspective and live our lives trying to mimic what we see on screen, creating our own relationships—with ourselves and with others—from this underdeveloped, profoundly empty baseline. This male-created portrayal breeds insecurity and dependency. As women, we are trained to look outside of ourselves for the answers and depend on men to rescue us. Even Belle from *Beauty and the Beast*, who was imprisoned and verbally abused by a man, later depends on that same man to save her—and eventually falls in love with him.

It's no wonder we are aching for something more meaningful.

In addition to being raised on cheap storylines and empty fantasies, I simultaneously witnessed this dystopian male-female dynamic playing out in real life in my own family, as far and wide as I could see. I observed women staying in unhealthy relationships with the belief that they had no other option. They should be thankful for what they had, they reasoned. At least someone chose them!

My "female training" should have included role models who helped me see possibility and a bright future. Instead, I learned from women who sought only to please their man with the next warm meal or perfectly ironed shirt. I wasn't surrounded by women who were hungry for a life outside of their constrained and miserable marriages. As I observed my only female role models, I began to wonder how my ambitions would ever fit into a traditional marriage. Even as an adolescent, I felt that ambition was a bad quality for a woman. That my dreams were too big, and I was too strong to ever attract a man who would want to spend his life with me.

I started to think that maybe I didn't know what was good for me; maybe I couldn't trust myself. Maybe the world knew better than I did. Maybe love from a man would be more important and more valuable than my own love.

Society sends constant messaging that women should prioritize love from someone else over one's own self-love. But that's a trap that keeps women needy and weak. We don't raise women to love themselves—quite the opposite. It's no wonder we become dependent on earning love, even if we're only getting breadcrumbs.

Eventually, I did meet a man who loved me completely and didn't hold the limiting beliefs I'd been raised with. But I still struggled internally. When I was newly married, my family, friends, and colleagues were more in awe of my beautiful marriage and my husband than of what I dreamed of for my future.

It often felt like I was a million miles away from my soul, in a world where my family was more interested in what I was cooking for a holiday than what I was birthing inside my soul. Their lack of understanding or curiosity about my passions was disheartening. There was even a brief time, when I was in my thirties, when I envied women who were less complex and ravenous than I was. It seemed easier to be compliant than compelling.

To this day, I've had to navigate so much around this from the external world, especially family. I have been made wrong for the fire inside of me, even by those who claim to love me. I've dealt with comments that I am too feisty, I take things too seriously, and I should be enjoying life more and working less. But I knew then, and know now, that I must honor my inner self—the Queen within me.

FROM BABY PRINCESS TO QUEEN

Like all women, I was subject to the indoctrination of seeking rather than being, of chasing rather than attracting. To illustrate these concepts and understand these operating energies in a woman's life, let's examine the archetypes of the baby princess and the Queen.

Let's first consider the baby princess. By "baby," I don't mean infant, I mean the princess's immature way of operating in the world. Like the archetypes we grew up with, the baby princess reacts to the world around her. She seeks approval from others, largely based on her beauty and youthfulness. She is fearful of the world, flailing about, waiting for a man to save her. She feels helpless but hopeful that life will get better, if only someone would rescue her. When the baby princess looks in the mirror, she criticizes what she sees. She knows her greatest asset is her face and body and hopes someone will sweep her up before her value diminishes.

A Queen, on the other hand, is rooted. She responds, rather than reacts, to the world around her. She knows the only approval she needs is from herself. While she understands the world fears her, she is still a helper, looking to lift others up. She curates her most beautiful life, and instead of finding value—or lack thereof—in her appearance, she knows her soul is what makes her special. She questions the messaging of the world, going inward for answers, always looking to fully engage in life.

In a world where the majority of women are brought up to *seek* worth, approval, and love, it's clear why women never fully develop the skills necessary to *feel* their inherent worthiness. How can a person become self-approving and self-loving when she's been taught that only others can bestow love and approval upon her? When I talk with my clients about filling themselves up with these attributes of inherent worthiness, selfapproval, and self-love, I am often met with furrowed brows and silence. Most have never even considered they could give themselves these feelings. Our patriarchal world has taught us that our worth is dependent on the man we are standing next to.

There is misery and emptiness in this patriarchal game. And yet most women continue to play along, believing they have no other option. To opt out would be the greatest failure as a woman. To be a good girl, one must never question the rules of engagement. Never.

After all, a woman who steps into her Queen energy is a danger to the patriarchy.

Even reading this book may feel like a dangerous opportunity because you can't unlearn what we're uncovering together. The choice is simple:

change your life or let your spirit die, as we see happening with all the miserable women and their addictions and illnesses. Speaking as a psychologist, the majority of medical issues are, at their root, unresolved psychological emotions. Women—including you—are suffering emotionally and physically, even if you think you are unaffected by the system.

Until now, we haven't had many alternatives. With few examples of women taking different paths, we look around and quietly take note that everyone else seems to have "figured it out." And while no one actually seems happy, many women resign themselves to the fact that unhappiness and submission must be the way of life. Keep acting. Keep having surface conversations. Keep accepting loveless or sexless marriages. Keep being miserable. Keep contorting and freezing oneself to fit a broken mold.

Eventually the mask cracks and many turn to drinking, shopping, overeating, and other self-harming behaviors. Alcohol, in particular, is one of the most accepted numbing drugs of choice, giving a false sense of pleasure that wears off as soon as the hangover sets in. This is such an issue in midlife that the National Institutes of Health conducted a meta-research study in 2022, in part to explore how to reduce harm for midlife women.[2] Addiction becomes a way to feel in control, to try and hold it all together, to not feel the truth rising. Better to hide one's true feelings at all costs, women reason. Medicate it away with wine or pills—but for goodness' sake, don't crack, don't feel anything, or you'll risk losing the façade of happiness.

Our culture raises us to believe we need rescuing. We must stay dependent and not stray. We must perform for approval and praise from our families and communities.

And when we play the part, we get the praise we seek. "What a good girl," they say. Replace "girl" with daughter, woman, wife, or mother, and you have the sum of what women are taught to strive for. A good girl is what society wants, after all—she's so much easier to control than a self-led woman. Women who are self-approving are too potent and unpredictable for our world to handle—too much truth-telling comes from their mouths.

Self-approving women, we learn, are dangerous. They may brainwash other women to behave the same way. These women are labeled crazy for stepping outside the programming. Deep down, society fears a woman who cannot be controlled or manipulated into a small and miserable life.

Society doesn't raise women to be self-sufficient. A woman on her own is thought to be a radical feminist, a spinster, or even worse: a societal failure. Examine your own beliefs. Where does your mind go when you find out that a woman you have just met is single at thirty-five or forty? The conditioning runs deep.

I hope, through our exploration, you see how you've been marinating in misogyny your entire life. You've been programmed to hate yourself and to please everyone else. And this awareness—this acceptance of reality—will enable you to move toward becoming the Queen of your own life.

Unlike the Queen, the baby princess is needy, relying on others to validate her existence and worth. She has fallen victim to the story that she does not matter—her life is worthless if she doesn't keep the man, the beauty, the youth. The Queen, on the other hand, deeply understands she has been brought up in a world with limiting storylines. She refuses to live under a spell. The Queen sees possibility and abundance everywhere. She understands, deep within her bones, that she is complete, whole, and safe.

A princess can step into Queen energy and change her entire life. Doing so begins with rewriting internal scripts and manifests through behavior change. Each woman must unearth her truth and rewrite the standards she lives by, no longer living life with a mindset of scarcity, a victim of her own distorted systems. As an example, one of my clients had been wanting to take dance classes for as long as she could remember. But her partner said it made no sense—she had no previous experience and most people had been doing the type of dance she was interested in for decades. Why start now? Through our work together, she stopped waiting for permission to live her own life, signed up for dance classes, and now travels the world with her group to participate in global dance events. Yes, Queen!

Another client found herself stuck in the mindset that it was too late to begin a new career. After further exploration, she discovered it was not her personal belief that she was too old to begin again; instead, she had internalized a worldview that wasn't true for her. As we worked through releasing this limiting belief, she was able to create an expansive energy and stepped into starting her own dream business—which is now not only wildly successful but has also brought her endless joy and freedom.

The women who go on to have the most phenomenal lives are not fixated on what is lost through aging; rather, they're focused on what is gained. They're creating masterpieces, learning new skills, having novel adventures, and seeing opportunities everywhere. They don't fear aging—they celebrate aging! They deeply understand that they are in constant metamorphosis, and they're excited to mine for gold in every stage of their lives.

A woman operating with Queen consciousness sources from within. She sees the limitations and lies society has built to keep women enslaved, the narrative that "your life only matters if you are chosen by another." No. A Queen chooses herself every damn day. That doesn't mean she rejects relationships, but her worth is not dependent on others.

Some of the most successful women I know see every nuance of life and every circumstance as happening for them, not to them. They see lessons and growth everywhere. They understand that the quality of their experience on this planet is determined by their mindset. Every day, every moment, we get to choose whether we want to be the baby princess or the Queen of our lives.

THE MIRACLE OF SILVER HAIR

During one of my trips to Italy, an American woman approached me in a restaurant bathroom.

"Your silver hair is gorgeous," she said, and went on to explain how she wished she could be brave enough to stop coloring her hair. She shared how her husband didn't want her to stop—even though he was gray—and even if she did decide to go natural, she would pay thousands to have a stylist transition her color in one appointment.

Encounters like this happen to me multiple times per week: in check-out lines, while walking down the street, and yes, especially in bathrooms. I've even given news interviews where the hosts focused largely on my hair! Time after time, I meet women who desperately want to be free but cannot fathom it for themselves. They stare at me as if I have a special superpower or magical secret I can share. And I can see they deeply struggle with my explanation: that I chose—I decided—to see my silver hair as an exquisite crown that signifies elegance, power, and wisdom.

When asked how I transitioned my hair from dyed to natural, women seem perplexed to hear that I simply stopped coloring it and allowed the gray to take its natural course. This is always the part that makes women's mouths drop open. They are shocked to hear I didn't cut it super short or color it silver in one appointment. It seems unbearable to them that I allowed, that I actually made the deliberate choice, to grow my hair out over the course of eighteen months, to witness the unfolding and becoming.

I wanted to be *in* the process of growing it out. I wanted to watch the miracle unfold before my very eyes. And most importantly, I was curious to see who I would become in the process, including the inner work I would have to do in this youth-obsessed culture. There are endless quick fixes in life, but they do not interest me because I know that I will not experience internal growth or change if I bypass the process of physical transformation. Every time I have walked the longer path and not rushed for the Band-Aid solution, I have learned so much about myself. My capacity to evolve continually expands during those experiences.

This is the consciousness of a Queen, a woman who sources never-ending invitations for her growth.

However, this level of conscious choice feels out of reach for most of the women I talk with. It's as if they can't believe that we, as women, can have that much agency over ourselves. That we can decide to anchor into any belief system. But we *can* decide. *You* can decide.

But if that decision feels out of reach, I can offer this hope: You don't have to love and accept the fact that you're aging before you begin to change. Instead, you can start by becoming aware of the conditions that have made aging feel so unnatural—as if it's something to apologize for. And as you become more aware, you'll notice, as a culture, most women care more about beauty than health. Again, we can showcase the baby princess versus the Queen: The baby princess relies on her youthful beauty for worth, with little inner depth; the Queen always chooses her emotional, mental, and physical well-being over the cheap lies and societal obsession with youth.

With the worldview of a Queen, you'll be able to see the beauty of aging: the wisdom gained, the life lived, and the potential still available. It's the victim who holds tightly to the way things used to be and cannot pivot to become the heroine of her own life. Seeing grown women running around acting like baby princesses is an insult to our divine nature as women. It's as though we've accepted that one's value declines with age. If you hold this belief, when will your daughter, or another young woman you care about, begin to believe it too? At what age will her value begin declining?

Instead, we must unlearn the perverse beliefs we were raised with in our youth-obsessed culture. We must reject the idea that our worth is connected to youthful beauty, and that an aging woman is disposable. Only then can we return to the ancient remembering that all beings are divine and holy. This realization holds inexplicable freedom—and that's what I want for every single woman.

It feels profound to live this way—unencumbered and joyful. Like you're engaging in the greatest act of resistance.

Yet I'm sometimes met with irritation from the very women I desire to help. They make side comments like, "How can you be so happy and free like that?" The subtext: How dare I be this happy and free without succumbing to the fear of aging and constant complaining about bodily changes? I've had to remove myself from so many spaces, conversations, and text threads with friends who just wanted to bitch about menopause, the changes in our looks, and the body aches. No thanks. I can't stand myopic thinking.

Yes, I recognize the shifts aging brings. I'm going through physical and emotional experiences too. But as the Queen of my own life, I've decided to see everything—and I mean absolutely *everything*—as an invitation to know myself better, to see what I am capable of uncovering, and to explore how much deeper I can take my spiritual practice of aging. I also trust my body's wisdom. Menopause is not a disease but rather a rite of passage into the next phase of life as a woman.

I decided to write my own narrative based on all I wanted to feel: freedom, new beginning, wonder, a deepening into myself. After all, a Queen creates her own story while the baby princess feels stuck in a prewritten storyline with zero agency over her life.

> *I've had to remove myself from so many spaces, conversations, and text threads with friends who just wanted to bitch about menopause, the changes in our looks, and the body aches. No thanks. I can't stand myopic thinking.*

But as I leaned into my silver hair and embraced aging, I realized I didn't want to take this journey alone. Where were the women who saw the world the way I did? The women who let their hair grow and their wrinkles deepen? Where was my divine sisterhood?

MISTRUSTING OUR SISTERS

Just as I saw few examples of healthy marriages growing up, I also saw limited examples of strong female friendships. If anything, I was bred with the belief that women could not be trusted. I was taught to not let other women get too close, because they might try to steal what I have: my man, my job, my entire life. As we've explored, these messages were confirmed in nearly every fairy tale, in which the evil older woman silences the princess, or the nasty stepsisters make the main character's life miserable. These stories taught us that women constantly put each other down and are a threat to each other's voice and safety.

Even today, instead of seeing sisterhood flourishing in our communities and on the screen, we are fed reality shows like *The Real Housewives* and other curated drama, all dangerous examples of women constantly hurting one another. And as you might expect by now, nearly all these shows, including *Housewives*, are created by men.

With these storylines, it's no wonder we feel threatened by other women. Infighting is all we are shown! And with these fractured, unhealthy examples of female relationships, women tend to then be even more dependent on their relationship with a man.

Funny, it's almost as if the system has been set up to keep women reliant on men.

When infighting or lack of trust happens in any group, the members become disempowered and cannot form community—and they certainly can't revolt against a system that serves to keep them down. It's the same with women. We are taught to not trust each other, to fear one another, and we begin to believe we have no access to sisterhood. It's out of reach. The only "safe" relationship is with one's partner.

This internalized misogyny is terrifyingly insidious. We rarely realize the impact distrust of other women creates within ourselves. The truth is it's impossible to be against other women and love ourselves, because the belief that women can't be trusted is an unconscious self-inflicted injury that prevents self-trust and self-connection. And if we can't trust ourselves, how can we build a life, listen to our intuition, or find our way forward?

This often shows up in the form of feeling threatened by another woman's success. Think about the last time you genuinely felt excited for another woman and her accomplishments. When was the last time you openly shared your achievements with others? Do you ever worry that your success may have others questioning you, wondering things like, "Who does she think she is?"

Women often play down their accomplishments and feel safer commiserating in pain. What could be possible if we instead learned to hold the frequency of celebration for one another? What if we learned to expect the same for ourselves?

Lack of trust in oneself and in other women leaves a clear option: the man in our lives. By internalizing the belief that men are superior, we default into putting all our energy into the relationship: listening to his opinion, making him happy, and seeking his approval rather than sourcing from within. Doing so causes us to miss the wisdom that women bring to our families, our communities, and our world. Defaulting to this relationship also creates hyper-codependence, an unhealthy, excessive reliance on a partner.

Too often we believe there is nowhere else to go—which is how it is for far too many women. And so begins the entrapment of staying in less-than-fulfilling relationships, rationalizing that at least they have a man, even if they're miserable.

In my work with women, I see this isolation happening everywhere. We've lost the art of gathering, supporting, and celebrating one another. We used to gather in rituals to have blessing ceremonies for periods, weddings, and births. Now we look to predominately male doctors for answers, for we have lost all connection to, and trust in, the body's natural processes. Periods, pregnancy, childbirth, breastfeeding, and menopause—women have been raised to fear these completely natural processes that have been happening for thousands of years. When asked about these particular stages of life, most women will speak about them with dread and annoyance rather than reverence and honor for all the body is capable of during a woman's lifetime.

As evidenced by my own experience and the experiences of almost all my clients, our mothers did not teach us about our phenomenal bodies.

If anything, we learned that our bodies were shameful, burdensome, and dirty. They taught us that we must deal with our feelings—fear, shame, self-hatred—alone, without the support of others. Instead of seeking support and connection, we hide behind our four walls and fences. This hyper-individualism is especially devastating for new mothers and has profound effects on the entire family system. Many of us believe that asking other women for help is too vulnerable; we'll be seen as a failure because we can't do it all. And besides, we reason, other women aren't safe. We fear our sisters because we've been taught by society and our female role models that women aren't to be trusted.

We have traded communing for competing. It's easy to control an entire group when they have been conditioned to distrust and be disgusted by their own bodies. It feels easier to put on a brave face and dye our hair than connect with each other. But when we reconnect to, and love, our own bodies and each other, we are unstoppable.

REFRAMING JEALOUSLY TO EMBRACE DIVINE SISTERHOOD

When we align together as women, we're even more powerful. Your joy and success have the potential to expand the scope of possibility for others. But how do you overcome the jealousy you've been conditioned to feel and embrace divine sisterhood?

Divine sisterhood is when all women hold respect, belief, and honor for one another and our lived experiences. A mindset of sisterly divinity desires to see all women thrive and knows that every woman's victory benefits the collective.

The opposite of this energy is the sisterhood wound, which is a deep patriarchal conditioning of distrust for other women and the belief we will not be accepted by other women.

Wounded women see other women as threats—it's the baby princess mentality that will keep us weary and needy. Our relationships with men become our world. The Queen, on the other hand, maturely chooses to align with other women and embrace their inherent gifts and talents. She sees the power in coming together. The baby princess competes but the Queen communes. While the baby princess has been brainwashed to believe in scarcity, the Queen knows there is abundance in all things.

In my own journey, life began to feel more joyful, supportive, and in flow when I leaned into sisterhood. Once I cultivated these relationships, I began to understand what had been missing my entire life. Sisterhood is the elixir, the north star, the place to be fully seen, understood, and honored.

I can understand how dangerous it must feel to the patriarchal world when women come together to share, support, and advocate for one another—and this connectedness is something the patriarchy will discourage at all costs. Such a community could completely destroy everything the patriarchy has built. Of course that's threatening!

I've witnessed the power of women speaking truth and deciding they want more for their lives. When women demand more from their partners, lives, jobs, and communities, it creates upheaval in a system designed to keep women suppressed. But when a Queen rises, removes the apology from her voice, and creates new standards for herself and her sisters, everything changes. Ultimately, what benefits a woman, benefits the entire world.

When we come together and start sharing our stories, we begin to understand and support each other. For there is no liberation for women if only a few are rising; we need millions of women awakening. We become stronger because of our numbers, and this volume gives us power. We can overthrow systems and demand better.

In order to create collective change, we will need to heal our sisterhood wounds and internalized misogyny, both of which are often passed down by our mothers. One's own mother is the first example of being a woman in the world—the imprint of how to be as a woman, and how to feel about other women. Igniting a revolution requires operating and relating completely differently from how we were raised. We didn't see examples of self-love and female friendships, so we need to *be* the examples.

Doing so requires engaging in new ways of relating to, and being in, sisterhood. One of the tools I use with clients is reframing jealousy. Most of us think of jealousy as a bad emotion, though it's normal to feel envious of others. But rather than feel threatened, you can instead reframe the trigger to become a treasure. Start by examining the thing you're envious of and asking yourself, "What does she have that I wish I had?" Is it a respectful relationship, a successful career, or impeccable boundaries? The answer to this question can inspire you toward action in your own life.

A common example I see in my work is women being triggered by another woman's comfort with her sensuality. When this comes up, I help women explore why this is so triggering and irritating to them. I guide them to explore the possibility that they have been raised in a world where women are not allowed to feel sensual, expressive, free, and whole in their bodies, so when they meet a woman who is all those things, it can be easy to make her "wrong." Once there is awareness of this, the real work begins.

These triggers are almost always invitations to what you are craving more of in your life. So rather than allowing negative feelings to take over, you can trade your emotions for a feeling of activation and then explore why you feel activated. In this case, you might discover you crave more sensuality in your life.

Once you've identified what you crave, I recommend three things. First, proximity. Get yourself close to women who are living the way you desire. Observe them, learn from them, ask them questions. Their energy will be contagious. Second, ask yourself where you learned that what she had or did was wrong. Where did you learn you cannot also experience that yourself? Where did your limiting belief come from—the one that says women should not behave that way or that only young women get to be like that? This part is critical in beginning to understand where the beliefs came from, and if they are even yours or were passed on to you through family, culture, or religion. Third and finally, make a list of all the ways you would move differently in the world if you had what she had. Once you have your answer, begin doing those things every single day. These daily actions will begin to change the way you feel about yourself.

Whether you're triggered by another's sensuality, confidence, relationship, possessions, or anything in between, know that you've been conditioned to feel threatened by other women; our brains unconsciously penalize others for their accomplishments. This can manifest through our thoughts and actions, such as making condescending comments in an effort to make ourselves feel better. Not surprisingly, this has the opposite effect. It's impossible to speak disparagingly of another woman and not simultaneously hurt yourself, for your harm toward them is also harm toward yourself and the entire female collective.

Who wants to operate at such a low frequency? Not me. By behaving this way, we miss the beautiful opportunity to learn more about ourselves and each other. But by instead trading the knee-jerk criticism for curiosity, you can begin to discover what you want more of in your life. Notice the power of your thoughts and words about other women. Allow them to inspire you—let them be examples of what is possible.

THE WORLD CHANGES WHEN ALL WOMEN SHINE

To put this into perspective, let me share a story I often tell my clients—the metaphor of candles at a party—to illustrate shining one's light in sisterhood. Let's say you've been invited to a party, and you bring a candle as a host gift. When you arrive, you see the host already has a candle lit on the table; you hand her yours and ask her to light it. To do so, she doesn't need to blow out her own candle. She doesn't have to say, "Oh, I already have light from my candle. We don't need yours." Instead, she can use her flame to light your candle, creating even more illumination. As each woman arrives to the party with their candles, the host can continue to use the already burning candles to light the new ones. Soon there will be a magnificent table filled with glowing candles.

The world changes when every woman shines brightly. Arm in arm, we rise together, illuminating the way for one another and all those who cannot find their way. Let us lean into the new narrative of being each other's sisters, way-showers, and traveling companions. Hand in hand, we will journey, each with our unique talents and medicine to share, for we need each woman to truly create a new way for all women.

Once we are able to self-approve and self-trust—to embrace our own humanity—we are able to trust other women and see their full humanity as well. The Queen has outgrown the outdated storyline the baby princess was raised on—the story of needing to be chosen, and approved of, by others. The Queen has chosen herself. She knows her own approval is all she's ever needed for her one and only precious life. She also recognizes life is richer in community with other Queens.

She understands that, in the natural order of things, we are meant to commune and share and laugh and heal and tend to one another. It is our intense individualism and isolation that are killing us.

I felt this isolation acutely as a new mom—and also the healing that sisterhood brings. I was profoundly lonely, as we were living in a new state, and I had not yet made any friends. My husband was traveling the world for work, and I was deeply craving community. I was fortunate enough to find a local moms' group and began hosting events for moms and babies in my home every week. I needed these women, this community: the sharing, learning, laughter, food, support, and safety of knowing I could share the highs and the lows with them and never feel judgment. All of us were new moms finding our way. Coming together was the healing balm for our hearts as our identities, bodies, and lives shifted dramatically.

We women need each other. By choosing to see each other as helpers and inspiration, we'll stop feeling fearful and threatened. We'll abolish feelings of scarcity. And we'll recognize that while we were conditioned to believe we are each other's competition, there will always be room for each of us to succeed. It's on us to see the truth—the manipulation and strategy that keep us at war with each other—and change our course forever. You can choose to mature from the baby princess who lives in fear to the Queen who sees abundance and love everywhere.

Women are holy, divine, majestic beings, and it's time to treat ourselves accordingly. We will not ask for permission from the patriarchy any longer. Instead, we'll define the context by which we want to live in, and contribute to, the world. And we'll grow our silver hair out if we damn well please.

I refuse to move through life as a victim. I refuse to adopt the shallow belief that I cannot create a beautiful next phase of life. I refuse to pass on a flawed model for my daughter, who is watching how I live and forming her own self-perception. Instead, I want her to see how I love my gray hair and celebrate life and aging with my friends. It's an honor and privilege to be a legacy breaker, to architect a new way for her—and all women.

From this place of self-love and interconnectedness, the next step is sacred. We must reclaim our physical bodies and tap into the wisdom of pleasure.

Chapter 7

RECONNECTING TO YOUR ANCIENT FEMININE WISDOM

"The most common way people give up their
power is by thinking they don't have any."

—ALICE WALKER

LET'S TAKE A lesson from nature. The acorn knows how to become an
oak tree by means of inborn essence. As the acorn takes root, if it's cultivated
in a nurturing environment, the new oak tree will flourish. The inherent
code for each next step is built in: seed, sprout, seedling, sapling, maturity.

An acorn contains a single seed within a hard outer shell, and within
that tiny seed is all the glory of an oak tree—an inherent blueprint of
becoming. And here's a fact that's especially interesting for our conversation: Oak trees become more valuable as they age. An English oak, for
example, doesn't begin flowering and growing acorns until it's around 40

years old. Its most productive years? From around 80 to 120 years of age. They can remain productive for 300 years, then live another 300 or more, serving a different purpose for the surrounding ecosystem, including as a continued habitat for other forest dwellers, such as animals and fungi.[1]

Like the mighty oak, every woman is an acorn, created with ancient internal feminine wisdom—at least until the world disconnects her from her natural essence.

Yet that perfect internal GPS system still exists within us. It can be excavated and revived. The female body is fascinating, and the life cycles of menstruation, childbirth, breastfeeding, and menopause demonstrate how intricately designed and miraculous our bodies are and what they are capable of.

The sad reality, however, is that girls are not raised by women who teach them about the honor and power of their bodies, including their cycles and how to support each phase of the month. There's a clear reason this knowledge isn't being passed down from mother to daughter: Their mothers didn't teach them. With each generation, we move further away from knowing how to listen to the wisdom of our bodies, to the point that we are fractured from, and completely unaware of, the mystery and power we possess within. This is tragic. As a society, we've almost completely annihilated reverence for the female body, except for what the patriarchy can use. There is no tolerance for anything that is inconvenient, messy, bloated, or emotional.

In the world of patriarchy, there is a solution for every "female" problem. Don't like the period? Take the pill. Don't want to use a condom? Insert an IUD. Don't want to feel the pain of childbirth? Get an epidural. Don't want to breastfeed? Buy formula. Don't want to experience hot flashes or hormonal fluctuations in menopause? Take hormones.

Notice how there is one toxic solution after another, all of which create huge profits. Every single one of these natural phases has been demonized, monetized, and marketed to, and worst of all, it's done under the guise of freedom of choice and feminism.

Compound this with societal conditioning to feel attacked or judged if someone chooses a different way—to birth naturally and avoid hormones and toxins. I've witnessed women simply sharing their experiences, only to be met with immediate shutdowns, shaming, and judgment. The result is that there's little to no room for hard conversations that can build momentum toward change. Only when we have open and honest conversations, within ourselves and with others, will we be able to fight the plague destroying our inherent existence as women and intimate connections to our true power.

TRUST IN YOUR INTERNAL GPS

This is true for all women, including you. But the onus isn't only on others. The worst insult you can receive can also be delivered by you: lack of self-trust. This manifests when you stop listening to yourself, when you completely shut down trust in yourself, and when you look to the outside world for the answers, rather than trusting your internal GPS. You were born with everything you needed to be able to blossom, including endless innate wisdom and divinity, and without connection to your internal GPS, you're now trusting in—relying on—patriarchy for the directions to your life. Since the system was written by men for the benefit of men, you can see how this becomes the most devastating blow to your entire life. And when your mother and every other woman around you sources from the patriarchy too, you can see how lack of self-trust becomes the norm for existing as a woman in the world.

I recognize that much of this information may be triggering you right now. So I invite you to pause. Take note of how you are feeling. From that place of awareness, I encourage you to look deeper. Examine the system that has removed honor from your natural systems. It's important to confront these triggered feelings. I want to always call us deeper, even—and most importantly—when it feels uncomfortable.

Discomfort can be a driver toward change. Allow it to push you to consider how taking direction for our female bodies from men who have never existed with a womb, and don't understand the inherent wisdom that it holds, is a destructive dynamic. From this perspective, it makes sense why we as women become so far removed from ourselves. Why we feel so confused, depressed, and resentful. It's because we have placed the control for our lives into the hands of men. Nothing could be more disempowering and diseased.

In this chapter, we'll explore how to reconnect to your internal GPS. By doing so, you'll be able to look inward to anchor to your inherent wisdom, rather than relying on the broken world around you. We'll get biological, detailing the beauty and science of key stages of the female experience: menstruation, birth, and menopause. And the first place to start is the place that is inherent to womanhood, your menstrual cycle.

THE CYCLES OF YOUR CYCLE

A young girl's first cycle is almost never met with celebration, honor, education, or a rite of passage ceremony. Instead, she is handed a maxi pad and told next to nothing about what is happening to her body. How profoundly sad and confusing. When women exist in a world designed for men, they learn to feel ashamed of their blood. Most women don't even know how to chart their menstrual cycle or support each phase with the proper nutrition, because it's not taught. As young women, we are even brought up to be grossed out by our own vaginas. We have been conditioned to feel inconvenient and dirty.

In the Old Testament of the Bible, Leviticus 15:19–23 (NIV) says: "When a woman has her regular flow of blood, the impurity of her monthly period will last seven days, and anyone who touches her will be unclean till evening. Anything she lies on during her period will be unclean, and anything she sits on will be unclean. Anyone who touches her bed will be unclean; they must wash their clothes and bathe with water, and they will be unclean till evening. Whether it is the bed or anything she was sitting on, when anyone touches it, they will be unclean till evening."

Many of my clients also grew up in countries that forbade girls and women who were bleeding from going inside the church. Regardless of weather conditions, they had to stand outside during the church service. It is no wonder they felt like something was wrong with them and internalized that shame.

Any quick visit to a local pharmacy will confirm these sentiments. Why is it that multiple shelves are filled with toxic products like douches, sprays, creams, and wipes? The message that women smell is unavoidable and belittling. Meanwhile, there are few, if any, products that exist for men's intimate parts.

Several years ago, I was at a restaurant with my daughter, and she needed to go to the restroom to change her pad. She asked to take my bag to conceal the package. I was happy to give her my purse, but I pulled her close and said, "Listen to me: You never have to feel ashamed about carrying a pad visibly in your hands. There's absolutely nothing to hide. Do you see all these people in this restaurant? Every single one of them is here because a woman had a period. Your body is miraculous. Hold your head high."

A few years later, I sat my daughter down again to discuss birth control. At that time, all of her friends were either getting on the pill or having an IUD put in. I shared the pros and cons of each, and how unnatural and detrimental each were for her body long-term, including her risk for cancer, decades of hormonal disruptions—even with the supposed "non-hormonal" versions that still disrupt hormones—and other complications. We also explored the health benefits of bleeding each month. Menstruation is natural protection against bacteria and helps regulate our vaginal pH; this self-cleansing process assists our body in protecting itself.

Menstruation can also be emotionally cleansing, a time to shed and release that which is no longer serving in your life. A time to purify, gain clarity, and have a deeper connection to your spiritual self. When approached with reverence, the experience can turn from dread to self-honor.

Ritual around menstruation is not a new concept. Before European colonization, many Indigenous cultures honored both first periods and monthly menstruation through ceremonies that involved dancing, flowers, singing, and ritualistic bathing. As we explored earlier, some modern-day tribes still engage in rituals that honor a woman's cycle.[2]

Personally, I do this through approaching the day I begin to bleed each month as an invitation to create ritual. I gather my most supportive items: candles, a heating pad, my coziest pj's, a warm cup of tea, my journal, and a pen. I allow myself to feel it all, to cry, to witness my emotions, to be tender and compassionate with myself. When I feel discomfort, I rock myself the way I would a baby. I sway my hips, get on all fours, and stretch my back. I listen to my body and intuitively follow her lead. This process has served my life in so many ways. My self-trust grows each time I honor what *is*, rather than making my menstrual experience something to "fix." And as I have learned to slow down and respect the power of my body as it does this most masterful work, I've allowed each bleed to connect me deeper to myself and my ancient wisdom.

In a patriarchal world where women do not get time off for their periods, I recognize that making space for this level of ritual and self-nurturing may be difficult to do. We need to advocate for fairer policies that support a woman during this time of the month. We are not meant to push through the pain and discomfort. That is highly masculine energy—the equivalent of "manning up"—and does not honor the female body whatsoever.

I mentioned earlier that most women do not understand their cycles. Self-education around our bodies is revolutionary, because the more we understand ourselves, the more we connect to our internal guidance system and start sourcing decisions from within.

Let's take a moment to consider just how powerful our female bodies are and all they are capable of in just one month—and continue to accomplish for years and even decades. In an effort to bring more honor to menstrual cycles, I strongly suggest becoming informed about each of the four phases of our monthly cycle: menstruation, the follicular phase, ovulation, and the luteal phase. There is ample beautiful information accessible for understanding the inner workings of our cycles.

Tracking your monthly cycle can also help you understand the why behind how you're feeling. Once you hold this level of knowledge, you will become better equipped to care for yourself in each phase and able to experience your cycles through the lens of self-love and nourishment rather than feeling gripping terror or disgust. In mature partnered relationships, you can also communicate that why, leading to deeper understanding and empathy from your partner as well.

It's clear that menstruation impacts our everyday lives as women, including our brain function. As an article in *National Geographic* details, MRI scans found that hormone fluctuation during menstruation "dramatically reshapes regions of the brain that govern emotions, memory, behavior, and the efficiency of information transfer."[3] Not that we needed science to tell us what we already knew, but the research confirms just how physiologically important these phases are. Understanding, and deepening into, one's cycle builds self-awareness and self-trust.

Of course, periods prepare us for the next stage: birth.

BIRTHING FOR THE PATRIARCHY

Like our cycles, the process of birthing—one of the most natural, innate female acts—remains a mystery. Our bodies contain the blueprint for birth. But just as with our periods, the act of giving birth has been profiteered and turned into a business. Rather than birthing from a place of deep intuition and self-anchoring, we are taking orders from the patriarchy. Instead of confident birthing, we birth from terror.

Medical systems sell fear so they can over-intervene during birth—the more procedures they do, the more money they make. The fact that the United States, a leading nation in medicine, has a C-section rate at 32.1 percent and rising is scandalous and points to how ill-informed women are about their rights.[4] Even more terrifying is that the United States has the highest infant and maternal mortality rates in the world, compared with other high-income countries.[5] How has something as natural as giving birth become so deadly? And why are women still allowing their bodies and babies to be in the hands of a system that sees them as sick and incapable?

Perhaps a more important question: Where are the counternarratives? There is little to no history of women and natural childbirth shared in our hospitals or homes. Women are not passing down stories of natural births but instead telling stories that perpetuate fear of our own bodies. We are so profoundly disconnected from our bodies, especially our wombs, cervixes, and vaginas, that it is not surprising we show up to the hospital, lay back, and let the doctors take over. After all, we have no context for believing we are capable!

When there is no history passed down about natural birthing, we believe it does not exist.

Here we can connect back to our earlier discussion of the vulva, because when we don't know our bodies—either anatomy or pleasure—we can't make informed decisions about our health care. There is an innate connection between orgasm and birth: the feeling of power, the sensuality, and even the guttural sounds. But we women have been taught to be ashamed of all of these, so it makes sense that shame carries into the birthing room. When you do not understand how to honor and work with your body—when you have been made to feel ashamed of your vagina and have never seen or touched your vulva—there is almost no way you can allow yourself the privilege and power of natural childbirth.

I wanted a different childbirth experience. Because I believed my body was designed with ancient codes and knowing for giving birth, I sought out a group of like-minded women and went to weekly classes with my partner. I also attended a weekly women's circle where I sat and listened, for months, to women telling endless stories of their natural births. Rather than the narrative of fear, I steeped myself in the most powerful, nourishing stories of women and the erotic nature of birth. And I read everything I could get my hands on about natural birth so that I was well-informed and prepared. Along with birthing classes, I joined my local La Leche League to immerse myself in all I could about breastfeeding.

The most powerful experiences of my life were giving birth to each of my children naturally, with midwives. I claimed agency over my body and my baby, I was informed and prepared, and I surrendered to the wisdom deep within. I understood that the pain was with purpose. I knew that if I listened to the pain, it had a message for me. With this knowledge, I allowed each contraction to guide me. During the birthing process, I was acutely connected to my babies, knowing that we were working together as a team.

Yet there was one moment in my first birth when the doubt crept in. I was in transition, the final stage of active labor where contractions are one on top of the other, each lasting up to about ninety seconds. This is the phase right before pushing begins. I knew this. I was prepared. And yet I had been in labor for fifty hours without any sleep and my mind was slipping into doubt.

Then, the most divine thing happened: images of women giving birth, all across the world, started to populate my mind. I saw women who were alone, partnered, in villages. And with every contraction, I harnessed the power of all women. I channeled their energy and started to feel a collective power rise within me. This was a pivotal moment in my life and a mindset that I still carry in my work today—that of collective sisterhood.

The experience of being in devotion to the natural birth process and honoring each phase was a warrior power unlike anything else I have experienced to date. The primal sounds that emerge from a woman who is feeling each contraction are similar to those at the heights of orgasm in lovemaking. Yet making these vocalizations can feel highly uncomfortable, as it requires completely letting go and merging with the primal process of bringing a human life into the world.

My first birth was completely opposite of that of most of the women I spoke with, and because I'd had such a life-changing birthing experience, I was inspired to help others do the same. Soon after, I became certified to teach natural childbirth and taught for ten years. I even cocreated a natural birthing app, iBirth, with my best friend, which has since been acquired by a prenatal company, supporting my desire to reach even more women around the world. The majority of my clients went on to have the most beautiful birth stories. When a woman did become fearful and gave her body fully to the medical system, she would reach out to me after and need intense therapy. Time after time, these women would equate their birth stories to feeling like they had been raped and tossed aside. Often, their sexual and bladder functions were damaged as a result of the aggressive interventions of the doctors.

These women's stories aren't unique—they're systemic. And harm to women's bodies and psyches can last for years. Even for the rest of their lives.

This is the truth. And yet I do want to acknowledge that I am grateful for Western medicine in the event of an emergency. However, that statement comes with nuance, because it's critical to understand that many documented "emergencies" are created at the hands of the medical system.

An entirely separate book could be written to detail how interventions often take on a cascading effect, with one spilling into another. One example is Pitocin, which is often given to a mom to "speed things up" by causing the uterus to contract. But giving Pitocin is like picking an apple before it is ready. The Pitocin often creates inhumane contractions that neither mother nor baby can withstand. These artificial contractions are nothing like the natural rhythm of a labor contraction. More often than not, the baby's heart rate spikes from the Pitocin and creates cause for concern, which can lead to a C-section to keep the baby safe. In many emergent birthing interventions, interfering unnaturally with the labor created the problem in the first place.

With awareness that women exist in a world created by men for men, it becomes clear that the act of childbirth is not supported in a way that is natural and primal for mother and baby. Telling a woman to lie on her back puts her into the most painful and unnatural position to labor in. The body is meant to be upright and swaying, which assists the baby in coming down the birth canal. A woman about to push is best supported in a squat, as doing so shortens the birth canal and allows more ease for both mother and baby. But the hospitals don't encourage or support this. After all, this position takes control away from the doctor. Instructing women to birth in a way that feels so unnatural feeds the storyline that women do not know how to give birth.

The birthing system strips autonomy and convinces women that they need saving from their own divinely created bodies. And we wonder why women feel profoundly disconnected from themselves, in birth and beyond. The first step toward shifting this fear is learning to trust your body, listen to it, commune with it, and see it as a constant, trusted advisor. When we educate ourselves about our bodies, we no longer fear them. When we no longer fear them, we are able to receive the messages they are sending us and work with them instead of against them.

I believe that when our wombs, ovaries, and breasts become sick and riddled with disease, it's because we are devastatingly disconnected from our feminine energy. Through rejection, suppression, and disconnection, we are contaminating our sacred vessels. It's just like when we pollute or try to control Mother Nature: the consequences of that harm never result in flow or harmony. With IUDS, birth control, and endocrine-disrupting personal care and beauty products, we have become far removed from feminine homeostasis.

I would like to suggest we turn back toward ancient practices of honoring our cycles, birthing experiences, and all the ways in which our bodies were designed so beautifully. I suggest we immerse ourselves into communities, both online and in person, that celebrate the feminine rather than dishonor and desecrate it. I've had to search far and wide to build my sisterhood of like-minded women. Yours are out there too. Sometimes it just takes a bit of time, but with intention and patience you can create a powerful support system.

All that said, I want to take a moment to normalize if you are feeling triggered or angry right now. We are unearthing a broken system that does not honor and protect women's bodies. It's normal to feel upset. Perhaps you've already given birth and don't see a point in revisiting what you can't redo. Maybe you haven't been through your birthing experience yet and feel fury that you now have to undo this conditioning or look knowingly away. Or perhaps you're thinking about a young woman you care about who will be going through birth soon, and you worry for her. I understand the fury!

No matter where your anger is directed, toward me or toward the system, I care enough about you and all women to keep sharing this information. We cannot look away any longer. Future generations of women need us to look right at the truth, and to boldly proclaim it.

When we as women begin to understand the power that resides within our bodies and how to work with this internal power, the collective will begin to reclaim and reconnect with our inner warriors and take back control of our bodies during the birth process, which is one of the most profound and life-changing rites of passage. This reclamation has the potential to shift a woman's entire life, in birth and beyond.

TAKING THE MEN OUT OF MENOPAUSE

A woman's period and childbirth are sacred experiences. And while there are many moments of divinity along the path of womanhood, the next big milestone is menopause.

I wrote earlier about my own experience trying to learn about menopause, and the endless articles that populated my search screen. I shared how I struggled to find details about the functional process of menopause, let alone how to move intentionally through such a critical rite of passage. During my search for a meaningful exploration of menopause, I found Darcey Steinke's work.

In her breathtaking book, *Flash Count Diary: Menopause and the Vindication of Natural Life*, Steinke details the extraordinary experience of studying and observing killer whales, the only other mammal that experiences menopause and lives long past reproductive years. She shares how the matriarch of the sea is revered and how the younger whales follow her around, learning from her. She questions modern-day humanity and the ways in which it overlooks aging women, and affirms menopause as part of a woman's natural life, not something that is meant to be treated with hormones and seen as a pathology.

Like with periods, let's demystify menopause. The root of the word comes from the Greek *men* for "month," and *pausis* for "a cessation or pause."[6] Medically, menopause is the end of your monthly cycle, generally in your forties and fifties, with the average age of fifty-one.[7] It is preceded by perimenopause, which can begin as early as your mid-thirties.[8] I detailed many of the well-documented symptoms of menopause earlier in the book, including vaginal dryness, night sweats, insomnia, and more, including the infamous hot flashes.[9] The main cause of these symptoms is a drop in estrogen levels—which is why pharma companies have rushed to prescribe estrogen to menopausal women.[10] You've officially completed menopause and are postmenopausal once you've had an entire year without a period, though symptoms can continue for up to a decade.

There is much more I could discuss about the physiological experience of menopause. Here, I want to explore the spiritual. In keeping with the theme of natural feminine states, I have also chosen to see menopause as yet another naturally occurring phase of a woman's life. Rather than vilify this stage, it should be honored.

Let me ask you: Do you actually think humans know better than Mother Nature?

Rather than fight biology, lean in. Decide to see this phase as a rite of passage and an opportunity to intentionally merge with your bodily changes. As in natural childbirth, natural menopause means you are no longer working against your body but instead stepping into the energy of curiosity around each change.

Estrogen levels drop because they are meant to drop at this phase of life. Why do you think so many women are unwilling to surrender to this truth? What are women afraid of? When we expend all this energy trying to recreate our younger years, we miss the lessons of now. We live outside of the magic. We miss the deeper invitation.

Worse yet, we're risking our lives. My own mother was diagnosed with breast cancer; after a double mastectomy, she was told that her cancer was most likely caused by hormone replacement therapy. I do not want to risk cancer by forcing hormones that are no longer meant to be in my system.

Personally, I want to experience the holiness of this journey. And now I am. During the final stages of writing this book, I stopped having my periods. As of this writing, it's now been five months without a period, and I'm in menopause at age fifty-one. And here is what I can tell you: I've decided to open to the journey and see who I become. And while I have not noticed any noteworthy changes—no changes in sleep, mood, sex drive, and not a single hot flash—I will walk with reverence into the changes to come. I will make menopause mean another sacred portal where I get to access parts of myself in ways never available to me before. When we remove fear from the storyline, when we recenter honor, the experience lands differently.

FROM MEDICALLY NUMB TO EMOTIONALLY ANCHORED

We've explored the core stages of a woman's changing body, from periods to childbirth to menopause and beyond. And we've discussed how to anchor intentionally into self-trust, access one's internal GPS in each of these stages, and make decisions confidently, rather than being passively knocked around by the whims of the patriarchy. Now let's talk about your feelings—those big emotions you've been taught aren't OK.

After all, the world tells us, no one likes an emotional woman. That's why we can't be in critical political positions. That's why we need a big, stoic man to keep us steady.

I'm here to break the narrative that emotions are undesirable. Instead, they are our superpower. Feeling one's emotions fully is critical to anchoring to your internal GPS.

With so many quick fixes and endless pills, deeply connecting with yourself and listening to your body from a place of honor has become a lost art form. But women have a vast emotional range; when connected to oneself intimately, a woman is able to express and emote, which is both necessary for daily functioning and also healthy. Our moods change just like the weather does—and this is a good thing! Strong emotions are not meant to be numbed with medication but rather witnessed like passing storms. When you begin to see your emotions as messages, you can use them to guide you to deeper intimacy within yourself. Feelings are the fertile ground upon which you grow your life. Be careful of a system or people who want to mute your expression.

Sadly, client after client has shared stories of being shamed for their emotions being "too much" or out of control, and feeling they had no choice but to go on medication. When medicated, many of my artist clients lost their ability to create, paint, write, and play music. Almost all of them lost their libido, gained weight, and overall felt numb to their lives. Many of them were convinced they needed their antidepressant or antianxiety meds to function, never questioning the havoc it was wreaking on their lives. Most of them were terrified to even entertain the idea of living without the medication.

When I helped them understand they were designed to feel, that their emotions were their guidance system, they got curious. Over time, I taught them how to live a more embodied life: to witness their emotions from a place of inquiry; to practice emotional hygiene rather than living in emotional dysregulation; and to use dance, self-pleasure, creativity, and nature as their guides. As they integrated these strategies into their lives, they were ready to fully feel again. The majority of my clients wean themselves completely off their meds because they understand their emotions were never meant to be snuffed out. It's thrilling to watch them reclaim themselves, hold more self-trust, honor their emotions, and have their libidos return.

With that said, I want to pause for a moment to acknowledge and celebrate that you are still here, still with me, and willing to explore these concepts. I know how deeply triggering a conversation around the perils of medications and other "fixes" at all stages of our female experience can be. With one in ten women ages eighteen to thirty-nine on antidepressants, as well as one in five women ages forty to fifty-nine, and one in four ages sixty and up, chances are you, or someone you love, is on a pill to numb these necessary emotions.[11]

> *The majority of my clients wean themselves completely off their antianxiety and antidepressant meds because they understand their emotions were never meant to be snuffed out.*

It's heartbreaking that so many women are walking around numb, going through the motions of life. No wonder each day feels mundane and "off." This place of discontent leads to excessive shopping, drinking, drugs, porn, and social media scrolling. Some women keep themselves too busy, overbooked, and over-serving so as to not feel. Most women don't even realize how deeply entrenched they are within the harmful patriarchal medical system and how it's actively robbing them of their true essence. With love, I am extending my hand in invitation to consider a different path forward.

And, Queen, you are already choosing a different path: one of consciousness. You've chosen to keep reading, which means you're choosing awareness. You're choosing to *see*. Being awake takes courage. Feeling in a world that tells you your own emotions are wrong and unsafe takes courage. You are courageous.

My deepest hope is that this discussion activates something within you, and from that activation, you're able to build a life that feels more aligned with your soul. That might mean working with your doctor to wean you off medication, assuming you have the support to access those emotions in a safe and healthy way. It's your right to live in holy alignment with your body, including its changes and range of emotions.

To reacquaint with your own emotions, you have to be willing to dig deep, get uncomfortable, and face truths and cultural assumptions you have been living your life by without ever considering why. This work will require you to listen to your body, sink into your emotions, feel for your truth, and stop betraying what your body knows is wrong. You must stop sacrificing your knowing to keep everyone else satisfied.

As I shared earlier, sometimes doing this work can feel like you are leaving family and friends behind. Often, speaking up or making changes in your life will cause those who love us the most to question our sanity. I have experienced this in almost every aspect of my life: natural childbirth, energy healing, business, medical choices, and so much more. When this happens, I have to lovingly remind my family that their fears are theirs, not mine. I tell them I deeply trust my body and I know what is right for my life.

I have been faced with parenting decisions that, for many, would have felt impossible, but my instinct is wise beyond reason, and I always trust my intuition to guide me.

Several years ago, one of my kids was facing some scary medical issues, including breathing difficulties. After consulting with a specialist, I made the decision to do the opposite of what he suggested. My son looked at me with concern and said, "But Mom, that's not what the doctor suggested."

I knelt down, put my hands on his shoulders, and looked into his eyes. "Has Mommy always kept you safe?" I asked. "Has Mommy always taken good care of you and your siblings?"

He answered yes to both.

"So I need you to trust me, my love," I told him. "And someday, when you are older, you will be able to trust yourself in these decisions."

It turned out my instinct to not put my son on a steroid inhaler and instead remove all dairy products from his diet turned out to be the exact remedy needed and completely opened his airways. These moments in which we model self-trust are incredible examples to teach our children to tap into their own.

Building on the exploration we've already done together in this chapter around our magnificent bodies and emotions, let's now explore the first steps toward living a life from a place of deep embodiment. Stepping into self-respect and self-reverence will be the pillars that support your journey when it feels too much.

QUESTIONS TO ACCESS YOUR GPS (INTERNAL GUIDANCE SYSTEM)

We've detailed how you have the most powerful internal guidance system. All women are born with one. The more you lean in and trust its impeccable ancient wisdom, the more you will learn to access wells of bodily remembrance. Even if you've lived a life without awareness and with self-harm, it doesn't mean your GPS has stopped working. Instead, it needs to be revived. You can relearn how to source inward for your decision-making, particularly when it comes to your own body. To do so, you must be willing to retrain the way you approach the relationship you have with your body.

This relearning process begins with self-inquiry; the next step is embodiment. When faced with a decision about your body, here are a few questions to ask yourself:

- Have I researched my options?

- Do I feel fully informed?

- Is there a story of fear influencing my decision-making?

- If so, where did that story come from?

- Is that fear actually mine?

- Can an alternative story be true?

- When I close my eyes, breathe deep, and connect with myself, do I trust myself?

- Do I feel capable and believe my body was made to be honored in all of its phases?

- Do I want to be in ceremony around this?

- How do I want to make this special, such as through creating rituals and new beliefs?

- Do I desire to write a new story for my legacy?

- Do I want to be the first woman in my lineage to reclaim her body and learn to lead with unshakable self-trust?

Inner questioning is the first step. The next step is making aligned decisions from that inner wisdom. Doing so will lead to a life of embodiment, which is what I deeply desire for all women. It's what I desire for you: to be connected to your periods, your moods, your symptoms when you feel sick, your intuition when something seems off, your ever-changing body and hormones. I crave for you to be in a symbiotic relationship with yourself, to feel every nuance of your intuition and to honor each as a message divinely guiding you. When you source from this place, you'll live with self-trust, peace, and a belief that your ancient wisdom is more sacred than any external quick fix.

Creating this kind of connection to oneself will require you to stop looking to the patriarchal world for confirmation, direction, and validation.

The system simply does not sell what you are longing for. On the contrary, the goods it sells will take you further away from yourself.

For a modern-day woman to live rooted in her femininity, to be simultaneously successful yet not a puppet to the patriarchy, requires the audacity to forge more beautiful ways for yourself and the next generation of women. Getting there requires intentional practice and a deeply grounded mentor to guide you on this path.

After engaging in this questioning, the next quest is embodiment. Embodiment is when learned material is no longer just cerebral information—it is integrated into your body and you experience it through your five senses. To begin the process of living more embodied, I recommend starting with the morning mirror practice that I share in chapter four. Beginning your day with meeting yourself in the mirror will become one of the most grounding and powerful practices of your life. Meet yourself with no critique and no objections, just pure love and reverence for what is. Feel awe at your humanity. When you begin to meet yourself as a holy being, holding space for the miracle of your life, over time your nervous system will begin to settle. You'll move from anxious and self-critical to wise and grounded in the majesty of your *beingness*.

Another incredible embodiment technique that brings you in alignment to self is dancing. This is not dancing to perform, to look a certain way, or to perfect a technique. Instead, it is dancing to *feel*. To connect to yourself.

Let me share my experience with how dancing took me to places within that I have never before tapped into. I've always loved to dance, but I'd never before taken any classes or danced other than out with friends, usually after a few cocktails, either at a house party or nightclub. Dancing was always fun but felt performative—always wondering how I looked while dancing. Did I look awkward? Repetitive? Weird? I had never fully surrendered while dancing, because I was too in my head and hardly at all in my body.

WHAT I LEARNED FROM POLE DANCING

Seventeen years ago, I was on a quest to feel more sensual, maybe even "sexier." As a busy mom, I'd put hardly any time or attention into my needs as a woman. My husband had been traveling the world for business for years, leaving most Mondays and returning on Friday evenings. There was a deep disconnect between us and it seemed we had little time to address the void. With my marriage in distress, and my husband and I leading essentially separate lives, I thought a pole dancing class might be the perfect remedy for all my issues. I joined a class run by a psychologist who was a former ballet dancer. I never could have imagined what was about to happen to my life and my connection to my body.

Through pole dancing, I started to discover a surrender, an intimacy with myself and my body I had never even known was possible. Every time the lights went down and the music came on, I felt transported into the most erotic and soulful places within. My movements were primal, and I moved in rawness, my dancing completely nonperformative. For the first time, my dance moves had nothing to do with how I looked. Instead, I was being led by how I felt.

There I was, dancing on and with a pole, an object and form of dance that has always been for the male gaze—and I was profoundly communing with myself and my body. The act felt simultaneously rebellious and sacred, and I knew I never wanted to stop. I felt a reclaiming, as though all the women in the class were taking back everything that had been taken from us: our bodies, our power, our sensuality. Everything that had been abused and commodified was being reclaimed every time I danced. I felt powerful. To this day, I am uninterested in technique or choreography; for me, the pole is the place I go to express, to reconnect, to be the rawest version of me, and I can't tap into that if I am thinking about the moves or my hand placement.

This practice helped my marriage in many ways, as I no longer felt resentment about never having time for myself. Instead, I claimed the time and took initiative. I felt more alive, sensual in my body, and turned on for life, which overflowed into the way I showed up in all aspects of my life, including my most intimate relationship with my husband. I connected to my femininity and healed parts of me that I had never before accessed, making me more fulfilled and balanced in our relationship. As I harnessed a previously unknown power within me, my confidence increased, which impacted how I led our family and our marriage in matters of the heart.

My clients tap into this deep self-connection too. I have one client who, every time she feels disconnected from herself or uncertain about her next steps, leaves her phone at home and drives to the woods. She takes her shoes off, hugs the trees, puts her ear to the ground, and listens. She breathes deeper. She lies on her back and looks up through the trees. She allows the magnificence of Mother Nature to wash over her and remind her that she, too, is as wise as the trees. All she needs to do is listen and feel, as her truth is within her.

When you're worried about the future or in regret about the past, it's difficult to source from an embodied place. Like I do on the pole, or my client does in the woods, bring yourself into the present moment, as this is where true embodiment resides. I make all of my decisions by feeling the answer in my body.

Embodiment is best tapped into through using your five senses: sight, sound, smell, taste, and touch. When in doubt about a decision you have to make, take a deep breath and ask yourself: What do I see? What do I hear? What do I smell? Taste? Feel? This exercise will move you into the present moment immediately.

With practice, you'll reach a point where you see, feel, and hear the truths of your heart—and wonder how you ever lived so disconnected before. You'll plug into your inner GPS to harness a deep connection with self.

This GPS also guides you into deeper levels of self-intimacy and sexual pleasure. After all, women were made for pleasure. We're meant to infuse pleasure into all aspects of our life. Consider this: A woman's clitoris has ten thousand nerve fibers, all designed for one single purpose—pleasure.[12]

Being in pleasure is a woman's natural state, but in our transactional, fast-paced world there is little time for pleasure. It is often seen as frivolous and ridiculous. Yet pleasure is the magic elixir to a beautiful life. A woman in pleasure radiates, impacting anyone who is lucky enough to be in her proximity. In the next chapter, I'll share with you how and why we need to curate pleasure every single day.

Chapter 8

RELEASING RAGE TO BUILD SELF-INTIMACY AND SEXUAL PLEASURE

"The body is like an earth. It is land unto itself. It is as
vulnerable to overbuilding, being carved into parcels, cut off,
overmined, and shorn of its power as any landscape. The wilder
woman will not be easily swayed by redevelopment schemes.
For her, the questions are not how to form but how to feel."

—CLARISSA PINKOLA ESTÉS, PHD,
WOMEN WHO RUN WITH THE WOLVES

MY PARENTS DIVORCED when I was ten years old. I was absolutely
devastated, overwhelmed with emotion, and uncertain how to navigate the
pain. Initially, I cried a lot and my family seemed to accept my emotions.

However, as the months passed, my grief seemed insurmountable, and my emotions continued to consume me.

I needed even more support and understanding, but the adults around me were growing tired of my tears. Their inability to help me led to feeling even worse, often resulting in uncontrollable sobbing. I was told everything from "you need to calm down" to "pull yourself together" to "stop being so dramatic." I started to feel like my emotions were a burden to my family, as though everyone was upset and impatient with me.

So, I did what most kids do to be liked: I stuffed my feelings way down inside of me and smiled, telling everyone around me I was fine. I swung drastically in the other direction and became the ultimate people pleaser in my family and at school. I loved the positive attention and all seemed to be going well . . . until a couple of months later, when I started getting debilitating headaches and unbearable stomach pains. My skin began peeling off in layers. And most disconcerting of all, I started to hear two very distinct voices in my head. One voice spoke with an exaggeratedly slow tone; the other, its archnemesis, spoke at a rapid pace and high pitch. The two voices bickered incessantly inside my brain. At times, the arguing was so all-encompassing I would be late for school.

Eventually the headaches and stomachaches became so intense that I couldn't even go to school. My parents, understandably concerned, took me to the Cleveland Clinic, where I had every imaginable diagnostic test run, including a full psychological evaluation. All the test results showed that I was perfectly healthy. In spite of the results, the psychiatrist wanted to prescribe medication to quiet the voices, but my father refused, a decision for which I am eternally grateful. We were sent on our way with a clean bill of health and zero answers as to why I was in so much pain. It's fascinating that none of those top-notch experts considered the divorce and my ensuing devastation as the cause—that my emotional turmoil could be the root of my troubling psychiatric and physical state. My symptoms continued for several more months, and I missed so much school that I started to feel completely alone and misunderstood.

MY BODY KNEW WHAT IT NEEDED

My mom knew something needed to change. One afternoon, she handed me a diary and told me I could write about my feelings in it. But even though I now had a tool to process my emotions, I couldn't bring myself to write my true feelings down because I was worried she would read it and feel hurt. Instead of processing my pain, I continued to exist as a sad lump of bones on my bed.

A few months later, now eleven years old, I became the proud owner of a record player, which I was allowed to keep in my room, and I felt the first spark of joy in a very long time. Little did I know my entire life was about to change. My first albums were all Lionel Richie. I distinctly remember the first moments, alone in my room, my door closed, the music turned up loud. As the lyrics to "Truly" began to play, tears spilled out of my eyes, and I bawled for hours. Song after song, I let the lyrics wash over me, and I felt the huge emotions moving through my body. This became my daily practice, and day by day, my headaches, stomachaches, peeling skin, and voices all dissipated completely. I finally had a way to let all my feelings move through me. I was no longer holding them all inside of me, poisoning my mind and body.

As I listened to the music, I wasn't just releasing my grief but also my anger and feelings of helplessness. Often, I would roll around on my bed, kicking, thrashing, punching, and screaming into my pillow. It brought such immense relief and connected me to my range of emotions without feeling afraid of myself. This practice became lifesaving for me—it was then, and has remained, the way I move my emotions through and out of my body. I now understand how wise my young self was to allow this raw and natural expression to evolve. I didn't make myself wrong for all my big feelings, and I no longer felt desperation festering inside of myself.

Accessing these emotions also opened me to discovering pleasure and my body. After releasing emotions, I would caress myself, which naturally flowed into self-pleasure. An entirely new universe had opened inside of me, and I finally felt free. I was sourcing from within, both by releasing pain and welcoming pleasure. My body knew what to do. It knew what I needed.

I was fully in my body. I was present with myself. I was no longer holding back or holding in but rather releasing and reconnecting. This healing process came from intuition, not from books or experts or advice from friends. I learned to trust the wisdom of my body, and my body's wisdom healed itself.

This is what I want for you: to learn to trust your body, to let it guide you to your own healing, to let your deepest wisdom open you up to the most beautiful life you can imagine.

Have you ever witnessed a woman like this? When she is fully in her body, fully being, fully present to the moment she is in? A woman like this is captivating. She carries an alluring, magnetic frequency that draws others to her. It's rare to meet a woman who is not anxious, posing, performing, or fidgeting under pressure. As we've explored, this is because, as women, we have become alarmingly disconnected to our bodies. If the baseline of interaction with our own selves lives in front of the mirror in objection and critique, how can we move through the world with presence and power?

Women are creative, destructive, beautiful creatures who have been tamed and made to feel crazy when harnessing the bigness of their emotions. As young girls, our wildness, mystery, and big feelings were squashed out of us. We learn to not trust our bodies—even to fear them and our intuition.

To live in your most divine state, you must be willing to reclaim your wild nature. After all, it is a spiritual reclamation to be a woman who trusts herself and her body. The body is divinely made and in constant communication with you. If you are willing to listen to the messages of your feminine body wisdom, you'll realize we have access to a superhighway of ancient information.

In this chapter, we'll explore how to reconnect to, and trust, the inner wisdom of your body. Embodiment is medicine, healing, the deepest connection to yourself. And if you actually want to be turned on, have a wet pussy, and feel desire, it is your job to get into this energy. The only way there is by creating a new way of being. You cannot do that from a lens of feeling "broken." And the first step to accessing your intuition: releasing rage.

RIGHTEOUS RAGE

Emotional regulation is a skill set anyone can learn and incorporate into their lives. I teach my clients the art of releasing their rage, desperation, and grief.

When I begin working with clients, and ask how they process emotions, they typically report that they talk to someone, meditate, go to yoga, drink, shop, or binge Netflix. Let's explore these and unpack how these methods are not long-term "fixes." Talking to someone about pain is a great way to verbally process and can allow for temporary relief and understanding of the issue. But this cerebral process keeps the pain tucked into a neat little controlled package that gets put back on the metaphorical shelf, never fully alchemized. I know women who have been going to talk therapy for decades with little result. They feel like they are spinning in circles.

Meditation and yoga, while both wonderful practices, were originally designed by men for men.[1] The practice of meditation is to clear your mind, to reach a calm and stable state . . . almost like you're completely ignoring the pain. Yoga is the practice of movements intended to connect the body and soul, to bring unity. But while these can be beautiful experiences, most practices are ineffective at reaching emotional catharsis. Emptying one's mind and lying in Savasana does not release rage out of the body. We also know that drinking, shopping, and endless television-watching are numbing mechanisms that take us away from ourselves and never provide anything sacred or healing.

Because we have been raised in a patriarchal society, we have been given patriarchal coping options. These methods are not designed for the feminine body and mind. As women, we are not meant to be still and silent while processing emotions. We're designed for movement. Dancing. Singing. Vocalizing. All of these practices enable women to root back into themselves and connect to their emotions. To feel the righteous rage fully and completely: scream, punch pillows, and let the emotions out. By using the movement of the body to alchemize the pain, we can feel it, honor it, and move it out of the body so that it no longer contaminates us. I like to think of rage as an erosive fossil fuel. As we dance it out, thrash it out, scream it out, we turn it into renewable energy that is good for our lives and the world at large.

When we look at the state of the world for women—the abuse, the objectification, the lack of rights, the silencing, all of which have gone on for thousands of years—we see how we carry unspeakable rage, both individually and collectively. Often, that rage is pushed so far down that we cannot feel it fully, but instead have a constant ache for a more beautiful life. That ache is safer to feel, and it can be numbed away each day through a few glasses of wine, or completely disassociated from through another meditation.

Alongside these societal traumas, many women also experience abuse in their personal lives. I recently received a letter from a woman who had been through deep childhood trauma at the hands of her father, and she had tried everything to overcome crippling anxiety, including suicidal ideation, that plagued her in adulthood. After learning rage-release practices, she got her life back. She was finally able to deal with her deep rage in a way that talk therapy and meditation never could.

In a world where women are conditioned to be pleasant and grateful, are called crazy or

> *When we look at the state of the world for women—the abuse, the objectification, the lack of rights, the silencing, all of which have gone on for thousands of years—we see how we carry unspeakable rage, both individually and collectively.*

unhinged if they show anger, and are told to calm down when they express upset, it's no wonder so many women feel disconnected from themselves—resentful and edgy. Rage is passion that has not been alchemized. We are enraged because the outcome we so desired feels impossible. We are enraged because we have been violated, silenced, abused. When a woman is sexually assaulted, the violation is so overwhelming it feels unbearable. Compound that with the fact that there is rarely any justice; if anything, she is left to explain herself and how she may have been at fault.

Women in these circumstances often retreat in fear and begin taking antidepressants or antianxiety pills, or both, to manage their emotions. What these women really need is a safe space to express their rage. They need to move the energy out of their body. Instead, they numb the pain because there are so few effective solutions to this kind of devastation.

And then there are women who claim to have no rage at all, and I understand why they are in denial. They're terrified of what may happen if they admit to their anger, if they feel or express the depths of it. I've worked with many women like this, and once they feel resourced with the skills to feel and move through their rage, they are shocked at just how much they had suppressed.

We have to stop looking away from our righteous rage.

As we commune with our deepest emotions and feel a sense of agency, we become increasingly more powerful, freer, and connected to our intuition. Clearing out the contamination enables hearing and feeling our deepest desires. Our truths. Simultaneously, we build trust with ourselves when we are not afraid of our darkness. When we can hold space for all of our emotions and usher ourselves, time and again, through the rage, grief, and heartbreak, we build a holy relationship with ourselves. It's similar to a young child who trusts a safe adult and knows that adult can receive all of their big emotions and not tell them to "pull themselves together."

Societally, we need to not just normalize adults physically processing emotions—we need to make it a regular part of our lifestyles. Catharsis has greater results than stuffing emotions down with food, alcohol, or endless scrolling. And releasing rage connects us deeper to ourselves and builds self-trust more than the male-founded practices of meditation and yoga.

Why all this talk of moving rage? Rage has a frequency, an energy, and when pushed deep inside, it contaminates our bodies, causing thyroid disease, autoimmune disease, chronic pain, migraines, and cancer. Rage also contaminates our relationships and bleeds onto others as resentment, anger, and impatience.

RAGE-RELEASE PRACTICE

I first learned about this rage practice when I attended an event hosted by Regena Thomashauer, and while I was shocked to see rage release demonstrated, I was even more impacted by the powerful experience I had when trying it for myself. I have since done the practice hundreds of times personally and lead all my clients through how to make releasing rage a regular part of their soul-care routine.

The practice of releasing emotions begins with setting the stage. It helps to have a playlist that evokes feelings of anger, loneliness, misunderstanding, and devastation, as such music helps support the energy needed to engage in the practice. I recommend having two separate playlists, one for grief and one for rage; that way, depending on the emotion you want to process, you will have what you need available. Often, processing grief can be an easier place to begin, and then you can move to rage right after. To support your experience, I've curated rage, grief, and sensuality playlists, which you can access at www.amandahanson.com/book.

Once you have your music playing, turn the lights down low or even off, with just a nearby candle burning, creating near darkness. You will want to be in clothing that matches your mood and allows you freedom of movement. I recommend stacking some pillows nearby, along with heavy-duty cardboard boxes that can be torn apart, industrial trash bags that can be shredded, or even old T-shirts and sweatshirts, which are good for tearing. Make sure the music is loud, the room is dark, and your supplies are within reach.

As the music begins, you may want to lie on the floor, slowly rolling side to side. Allow yourself to tap into your pain, your grief, your hurt, your isolation, your memories of being mistreated, misunderstood, used, abused. Do not force but rather *allow*. It may take a couple of songs before the feelings are accessible. As the feelings arise, you can begin to imagine you're showing the world what the pain "looks" like. Let your body move in the most raw and primal of ways. Shake your four limbs aggressively, stomp your feet, punch pillows, tear into fabric, and allow the resistance of the material to fuel your expression. Screaming, howling, guttural moaning are all incredible tools to move the repressed energy out of your body. There is no wrong way to express yourself. Just allow your body to move instinctively.

If the music ends before you're ready to stop, you can restart the playlist and continue releasing until you feel complete. After releasing your emotions, I suggest dancing to a sensual song afterward. This step is important to finish the practice fully back in your power. You have just released high amounts of energy, and dancing to a sensual song resets the tone and energy within. You'll end feeling powerful, with self-ownership—similar to the phoenix rising from the ashes.

Don't be alarmed if you notice your body trembling after this practice. The release of heavy emotions is a big energy to move and you will feel the release in a variety of ways, including fatigue. Many of my clients have also reported feeling energized immediately after. You'll have your own perfect experience, meant just for you, and each time will be unique. Trust the process and do not be afraid of darkness, ever. It will not destroy you. But holding rage inside and trying not to feel it very well may.

This practice may feel awkward the first few times, and you may notice yourself in your head, overthinking or judging yourself. This is normal. Be patient. Learning to hold space for your dark emotions is a practice that may take a bit of time—after all, you've been taught to suppress emotions for decades. Most importantly, remember there is no wrong way to engage in this practice. Let your body guide you and return to this practice over and over again as an honoring way to move dark energy out of your body.

OPENING UP TO SEXUAL PLEASURE

We have explored the ways in which we have become further disconnected from ourselves around the natural cycles of life, and how we have been conditioned to not feel our emotions fully. Now let us take a journey into female pleasure. In the context of patriarchy, female pleasure has been owned by men, for their pleasure and use.

The dominant messaging around sex in the world is that it is for the male gaze, enjoyment, and profit. From strip clubs and pornography to threesomes and sex clubs, we have been socialized to view pleasure through the lens of what men want, and society has left very little room for women to express their desires. Often, when a woman does communicate how she wants to be pleasured, she is called loose, a whore, or a slut. Male pleasure is often aggressive, dominant, demeaning, and focused on the goal of orgasm.

Female pleasure, on the other hand, is stoked when all five senses are engaged and heightened. A woman in her most sensual state is not performing, rushing, or focused on the outcome. A woman is lost in the art of the exchange, the pleasure, the sensations. Those experiences alone can activate and fulfill her for hours. But our fast-paced, masculine, goal-oriented world has not allowed the spaciousness required for women to be in these heights of ecstasy. I'm certain the fear of vulnerability is what keeps most people from engaging in slow sex.

This is not an issue of women not liking sex and pleasure; it's an issue of feeling incredible shame if we express our true desires. It's an issue of allowing patriarchy to lead the narrative and for porn culture to dictate the norms.

It's even more insulting when porn is used to measure female arousal—such as in the Netflix show *You Are What You Eat*, which attempts, among other things, to prove that vegan diets increase female sex drive. The deeply flawed study, run by Stanford University, compares sets of twins over an eight-week period as they follow either an omnivore or vegan diet, and tracks success through markers like body weight and LDL cholesterol. They measure sexual arousal by having each twin choose a flavor of porn, then having them masturbate as the camera pans out to a closed door, where the viewer is left to assume they are orgasming. Not only is this method of study deeply disturbing, but it further makes the point that pleasure for women is measured by a cheap tool—visual images, porn—used by men for arousal.

I learned later that Stanford didn't even include sexual arousal in their study. According to the lead researcher at Stanford, Netflix added this measurement without his knowledge—and he only found out about it after the screening.[2] Can you imagine being one of those twins, having your orgasm measured in front of millions of people, only to learn it was all a ploy for titillation disguised as science? Not only that, but for the doctors involved in that portion of the "study" to assume that porn would be the most effective route to gathering arousal data . . . well, it just shows a limited capacity to think women could ever be turned on by anything more. This is a perfect demonstration of the profound ignorance in regard to female pleasure and why countless women report how disconnected and unenjoyable their sex lives with men are.

The patriarchy's definition of female pleasure leaves the average woman completely unsatisfied and disconnected from her desires . . . and, eventually, completely numb. This lack of understanding, and valuing, female pleasure is why so many women eventually stop having sex with their partners: it is monotonous, uninspiring, transactional, and predictable. When couples use porn as the gold standard, it becomes clear why there is a massive void to understanding what women truly long for.

Client after client has shared stories of needing to have a few drinks before they can have sex because they feel so uncomfortable in their bodies. Many do not feel safe being completely vulnerable and have never felt safe in their bodies.

Let me repeat that: Many women have *never* felt safe in their bodies.

There are multiple reasons for feeling a lack of psychological and physical safety. Some women shared about past sexual violence or trauma; others shared that they have not spoken up about their sexual needs and have gone along with things that didn't feel good to them. The latter often happens because women have been conditioned to believe they have to "give it up to their man" to satiate his primal needs. This is a dangerous storyline to perpetuate and keeps women feeling used and unseen during intimacy.

A connection to your body and your pleasure is something you must reclaim if you are to ever feel completely liberated. In my practice, I have seen that disconnection from true sensuality is at the root of endless suffering for women and their relationships. Women are trapped in a circus of cheap distractions, unrealistic ideals, and unreachable images of what men want. Afraid and uncertain how to traverse the world of sexuality, sensuality, intimacy, and sex, many stay trapped in sex that is nothing more than robotic mutual masturbation.

As the desire grows for something more erotic, so does the likelihood of an affair. But even when women do seek a new partner, the passion and newness dwindle after the initial six months, and the search begins again. This cycle perpetuates because women are actually searching for something much deeper. Most are not even aware of what they truly desire: profound sensual connection that goes well beyond momentary great sex. They crave the kind of sensuality that pierces the soul and renders one completely speechless, overflowing with pleasure.

To build lives of rapture and pleasure, you must be comfortable in your own body. You need to define your own set of standards and desires, and stop accepting the violent, porn-driven definition of pleasure, as it will never allow vulnerability and erotic passion to build. To build a life of pleasure, begin within.

In my work with women, I teach self-intimacy and exploring their phenomenal bodies—their intricate and unique landscape. It's astounding how few truly understand not just their anatomy, but also the power they carry within their female bodies. I teach women about the art of turn on, strip tease, pole dancing, self-pleasure, crystal dildos, and much more. The fascinating thing is that I teach these concepts through the intention to connect deeper with oneself. Most women have never considered any of these things for themselves and have only ever understood sexual intimacy through the male gaze. No surprise there.

When you finally decide to stop being in princess energy around your body and pleasure, you can step into Queen energy and build sacred intimacy with yourself. Your pleasure waits for no one. Stop waiting for direction to your own joy and go on your own treasure hunt for what turns you on.

Pleasure is your birthright, but in this hustle and grind culture, we have become far removed from how to access pleasure. There seems to be no time when we are rushing everywhere. Consider this: Which females in your life role-modeled pleasure? Who did you see taking time for themselves, indulging in long walks, hours of poetry under a tree, gathering with friends around the fire for soulful conversations? Pleasure is about giving yourself attention and nurturing your soul. It's the little additions to your daily life that make it feel extra special, from lighting a beautiful candle while daydreaming to dancing in the mirror for yourself. Pleasure is sensual fulfillment for a Queen.

ADD PLEASURE TO YOUR DAILY LIFE

Pleasure isn't just about sexual fulfillment. In fact, you can add more pleasure to nearly every moment of your day. Get really creative with how you can infuse pleasure everywhere and notice how you begin to feel. Look for ways that you can feel more joyful, peaceful, centered, sensual, alive, and spacious.

To start building your pleasure list, ask yourself how you can add pleasure to your everyday life, including spaces like your bedside table, desk, car, home (bathroom, kitchen, family room, bedroom), music playlists, or home library. Consider the activities you do during the day and how you can add pleasure getting dressed, preparing meals, doing meetings for work, carpooling, doing laundry, or washing your face. Think about sexual intimacy too: self-pleasuring and having sex with your partner. As you add in more pleasure to different areas of your life, keep layering it into everything you do and watch your life transform!

Pleasure can be found in surprising ways, and in surprising places. There was a long period of time in my life during which I could be found in my laundry room until the wee hours of the morning. Kids and dogs meant never-ending laundry in our home. On a typical weeknight, with my children all quietly tucked into bed and my husband away for work, I would walk into my laundry room for another date night with the piles of clothes that needed TLC—tender loving cleaning. As you might imagine, this started to feel monotonous and exhausting.

One night, while standing in my laundry room, I wondered: How could I possibly make this space and experience more enjoyable? I started to daydream of lavender cabinets, crystal drawer pulls, a petite chandelier with a dimmer, candles, a countertop speaker, and a teapot. I had a vision of being enveloped by the space every time I stepped in. I could see, smell, hear, feel, and taste the space. Now it was time to take action and bring the laundry room alive. And I did!

When the space was complete, I stood back to marvel at the difference. These minor additions not only transformed the room visually but also shifted how my body felt when I stepped inside. Rather than dreading my daily laundry task, I started to look forward to it!

There are opportunities to infuse pleasure everywhere in our lives. Have fun with this mindset, and see how open and creative you can get.

BUILD INTIMACY WITH YOURSELF

Often, the word "intimacy" is equated to being intimate with someone else. Similarly, emotional and physical intimacy is considered a shared experience. And while that is a beautiful perspective, I believe it is paramount that we first take time to deeply travel within, to take a journey into ourselves, to learn how to craft self-intimacy. When teaching this concept, I have my clients take a look at the following list and circle all of the qualities they desire in partnership, whether a lover, a close friend, or family member.

- Trust
- Safety
- Joy
- Compassion
- Vulnerability
- Curiosity

- Patience
- Understanding
- Devotion
- Honor
- Tenderness
- Unconditional love

Often, we desire many of the above qualities to be fulfilled in relationships; we have learned to *seek* what we desire rather than *be* what we desire. Of course, human beings are made for relationships with others, but there is a difference between communing with another person and being heavily dependent on others to meet all our needs. For example, many women want their partner to honor them. That's fantastic, and I agree partners should honor each other. But self-honor comes first. When my clients share a desire for honor, I explore this with them by asking: How much, and how often, do you honor yourself? They typically look at me as if I have asked a trick question.

Most women don't know how to meet their own needs and expect qualities like unconditional love, tenderness, and curiosity to come from outside of themselves. Because of this, women become not only dependent on others for their functioning but also often trapped in poor relationships because they are unable to source their emotional needs from within. This lack of emotional self-sourcing is a huge deficit I see in most women. Once you learn how to source from within, you'll not only be able to teach someone how you like to be treated, but you are also so much more enjoyable to be in a relationship with because you're not exuding a desperate, needy energy—which, over time, becomes suffocating and unenjoyable to be around.

After defining the things you desire in a romantic relationship, ask yourself this question: Do I give myself _____? Go through each quality in the previous list one by one, answering this question honestly.

As you do so, notice which qualities you deprive yourself of. Notice how you long for certain qualities from others but are unable to give them to yourself. Notice how not meeting your own needs creates a seeking, a desperation, a neediness from others . . . the energy of the princess. A Queen sources from within, which makes her energetically magnetizing because she does not enter relationships from dependency but rather from fullness and overflow.

Crafting intimacy with oneself is a skill that will nourish every aspect of your life.

To begin developing self-intimacy, imagine you are just meeting yourself for the first time. You're on a first date and just getting to know yourself. What would you want to know? What questions might you ask? Feel free to add to the following list.

- What music do you love?
- What makes your heart break?
- What do you regret?
- If you could have dinner with anyone in the world, who would it be?

- If you had millions of dollars to donate, where would you send the money?
- Who is your favorite poet?
- What is the mantra you live by?
- If you were stranded on an island and had only one food for the month, what would it be?
- Who is your favorite actress, and why?
- What terrifies you?
- What has caused you the most pain in your life?
- What is the one thing you are most insecure about?
- What makes you laugh until you cry?
- Who do you dream about?
- What is the one quality you fear is unlovable?
- What do you do with your grief? Rage? Love? Overwhelm?
- What is your biggest turn-on?

Once you've gotten to know yourself better, you can continue to deepen self-intimacy by asking the following questions.

- How do I comfort myself when I am upset?
- How do I speak to myself when I make a mistake?
- How do I view my body?
- What do I do to celebrate myself?
- What is my favorite form of self-touch?
- How do I pleasure myself?
- When I want to feel seen, what do I do?
- When I want to feel heard, what do I do?
- When I want to feel cherished, what do I do?

- When I want to feel romantic, what do I do?
- When I want to be seduced, what do I do?
- When I want to be orgasmic, what do I do?
- When I want to feel like the most incredible woman, what do I do?

By understanding the answers to these questions, you'll be able to uncover areas to focus on and grow your own self-intimacy. Everything shifts when you expand and deepen your connection with yourself. Learning to source from within is one of the most powerful tools available to you, and deepening self-intimacy has transformed the lives of the majority of my clients. It can for you too.

As we've explored, we are not taught how to develop intimacy with ourselves, and doing so can feel uncomfortable at first. But like anything else, over time and with practice, you will begin to deepen into the landscape of your emotional and physical body, and you'll be astounded at how available that connection is—and has always been.

I want to lovingly remind you that the goal in life is not happiness. Instead, the goal is to feel it all, to let the wide range of human expression and your humanity be honored, expressed, and seen as holy. You do not need to be afraid of yourself, your rage, your darkness, your body, or your sensuality. You were made divine and all of you deserves to be seen. The journey to self-intimacy begins with truly meeting yourself.

Chapter 9

THE GRATITUDE TRAP

"In becoming forcibly and essentially aware of my mortality,
and of what I wished and wanted for my life, however short it
might be, priorities and omissions became strongly etched in
a merciless light, and what I most regretted were my silences."

—AUDRE LORDE, *SISTER OUTSIDER*

SEVERAL YEARS AGO, when daily gratitude practices like nightly journaling became all the rage, I watched countless women implement gratitude practices into their lives. At first, I thought this movement was absolutely beautiful. Along with the intangible benefits of living a grateful life, gratitude practices have been shown to increase happiness, reduce inflammation, improve sleep, and reduce anxiety, among other health advantages.[1] There are endless positive benefits to practicing gratitude! That's why I am a gratitude devotee.

However, I soon realized being grateful is only half the conversation. Yes, writing down all the things you are grateful for that day, and in your life in general, is a powerful practice. And yes, it expands your ability to acknowledge all of your blessings. Yet more can be added to this practice to make it even more profound and impactful.

Consider the last time you were in conversation with someone, sharing a hardship you're going through. Did they witness your experience through listening and reflecting back your feelings, making you feel seen, supported, and validated? Or did they rush to remind you that "it could have been worse," or "at least you don't have it as bad as most," or the most cringe-worthy, "you have so much to be grateful for." While most people are well-meaning, stating the obvious can feel like a complete erasure of what you were vulnerably sharing. Such comments create a disconnect in the relationship.

Now, another question: Have you ever done this to someone else? We all have, myself included. Next time, instead of rushing to focus on gratitude, pay attention to the nuances of human language, interaction, and reciprocity.

Sharing struggles with others is partly an attempt at building connection and partly laced with unspoken desire: what you wished would have happened or would have been different in the experience you're sharing. When the listener points straight to gratitude, it can feel like there is no room for duality. We can be upset *and* we can be grateful. We can struggle *and* be thankful. But when someone points straight to gratitude, the sharer can feel guilty for even thinking the challenge was that big of a deal to begin with. I see this play out for women over and over in their relationships, both with friends and partners.

Circling back to the gratitude journaling craze, I saw this trend take off almost exclusively with women, and the lack of male participation got me curious. I started to wonder: What would happen if women started a desire list? What if women were to draw a line down the middle of the page; one half of the page is everything they are grateful for, and the other half is everything they desire. I wondered: Would gratitude be the longer list?

I put my curiosity to the test and had dozens of women in my next workshops create their lists. The results were astounding. Just as I had expected, the side for gratitude was full. Women often even used the middle of the page to write more! In sharp contrast, the desire side was completely blank for almost all of the women. Why was this the case?

At one workshop, I had thirty women, ages twenty-eight to sixty-five, go around the room one by one, sharing their lists. Each of them enthusiastically shared what they were grateful for, but when it came to their desires, most lists were blank or only listed a couple of uninspiring things, like a nap or a clean garage. A few of them cried and shared they had zero clue what they desired. Many reflected that nobody had ever asked them what they desire in life. One woman said she has no time to desire; another said she knew what her husband and children desired, but not herself. Some said desire is pointless, while a few others stated they were too tired to desire anything.

Sitting with these incredible women, listening to them struggle to desire anything profound for their lives, was simultaneously sad and enlightening. Finally, I was tapping into the beliefs women carried about desire. The experience was also personally clarifying, because I was finally able to identify why the gratitude practice alone was so off-putting to me—why it had felt off all these years.

Many spiritual traditions also proclaim that we should let all desires go, as they keep us from living in the present moment. The Bible states that sin is born from desire. I am sure these messages have also played a part in making many feel gluttonous or wrong for having desires. Layer in the time scarcity many women experience as the main caretakers of children, family scheduling, and the home, and it makes sense that women are too exhausted to think about what they want.

I've since led many more workshops, each of which confirmed that women are already filled with gratitude, maybe even to a fault. It's not lack of gratitude that's the problem—it's a desire deficit hindering them from living more beautiful lives. From this experience, and many other workshops and conversations, I found that the art of gratitude is an exquisite and soulful practice in awareness, but it is only half of the equation in the human experience. If we are to truly feel alive, we must be grateful *and* desirous. It's not either/or, it's both/and. The combination creates the feeling of butterflies and excitement that bubbles up from deep within.

In this chapter, we'll explore the problem of toxic positivity and how it robs you of desire. We'll work together to identify what you desire and bring that desire into your everyday life, decision-making, and relationships. And building on your inner wisdom, you'll tap into your body's knowing, what your soul craves, to uncover the desires that will help you live the life of a Queen.

TOXICALLY POSITIVE

Women have been tamed into toxic positivity and over-giving, leaving little space for awareness of their own desires. It can even feel selfish and childish to desire more for your life. Many women worry that if they crave more, and vocalize their desires, they will be vilified. After all, isn't self-sacrifice the epitome of a good wife, daughter, mother, sister, and friend? I've even had clients tell me that, when they did share their desires with their partner,

> *If we are to truly feel alive, we must be grateful and desirous. It's not either/or, it's both/and. The combination creates the feeling of butterflies and excitement that bubbles up from deep within.*

they didn't receive support. Instead, the partner got defensive and made it all about themselves, saying things like, "Oh, so our life together isn't enough for you?" and "You need more? More of what, exactly?" and "You're never happy."

Gratitude and toxic positivity become traps when they are used for coping and repressing feelings. Often, when a woman is uncomfortable feeling the ache of desire, she copes by slapping on layers of gratitude. When she longs for a deeper connection in her relationship, she reverts to all the positive things about the union so as to not feel the pangs of emptiness for what she truly desires more of in partnership. Women spend most of their lives living this way, denying themselves the beauty of what they are ravenous for. Many do not even believe they deserve their desires because they've been socially conditioned to be knee-deep in gratitude. That if they desire more from their lives, they are unhappy and ungrateful.

We must normalize holding duality—that two things can be true at once. You can both love your life and want more for your life. One does not negate the other. When did we stop allowing expansiveness and abundance to feel like our birthright?

I've met endless clients who have checked all the boxes on the patriarchal checklist and yet still feel a constant, haunting ache. They have the career, house, partner, children, financial stability, and all the things they were told would make them happy, but the ache persists because what women desire is typically not the things they were told would make them happy. Instead, they crave the beauty and magic of life. The connections, the depth, the meaning, the sacredness, the romance.

I'm on a mission to awaken as many women as possible into discovering their desires. In my decades as a psychologist, I've seen too many women who have given up on themselves and their dreams. By the time they come to me, their internal light is dim, almost about to burn out. They are no longer thriving but simply surviving in a life that has very little spaciousness to experience anything outside of their to-do lists.

A first step to access desire for them, and for you, is to dig into early childhood memories. To recall all of the ways you played and created imaginary lands. When you were a young girl—seven, eight, nine years old—what did you love to do? If someone went looking for you, where would they find you? What activity would you be engaged in? What was that one thing you could get lost in, forgetting about the world? That activity you were so engrossed in that hours passed without you realizing it? Where you were full of joy, consumed in the magic of it all?

My clients recall climbing trees, playing veterinarian, painting rocks, dancing around the living room, building forts in the backyard. Each of those memories would then be translated into what they desire today. My client who loved to climb trees joined a local hiking group. The one who played veterinarian now volunteers at a dog shelter one day per week. My client who painted rocks has turned a spare room in her home into an art studio where she paints daily. Dancing around the living room has turned into taking salsa lessons. The client who built forts in her backyard rediscovered her love for camping.

If you don't know where to begin, ask your younger self to take you back down memory lane, because it's likely where your desires are waiting to be rediscovered. As you do this inner work, it will be essential to not allow excuses and logic to creep in. After all, there is absolutely nothing logical about desire. That's what makes it so special and why we feel fully alive when we live into our desires! Life is not meant to be just a list of to-dos; pay close attention if your life has morphed into that. What can you do to infuse windows of time for playfulness, for dancing, for desires to be fulfilled?

Make sure to stay in Queen energy here, because it can be easy to slip into victim energy and see no solutions for your life. Desire is your soul wanting to express that which lights you up from within. And here is what is even more incredible: Living into your desire benefits the world. Your expression, your art, your joy, your creations are gifts to everyone who gets to interact with or experience your unique expression.

Many women even try to delude themselves into a life of contentment, to convince themselves that their lives are satisfying enough. They don't allow desire to be felt for long, because desire can feel like a threat to contentment. Our female contentment conditioning runs deep. And as we've explored, when we have few examples of women claiming more for their lives, we believe more is inaccessible.

When we do crave more, we often stay quiet, trying to talk ourselves into being happy with what we have. Not rocking the boat. This often comes from a well-meaning place: We don't want to threaten or trigger another woman by desiring more. So we keep our desires quiet, barely admitting them to ourselves, and eventually talk ourselves out of wanting something greater for our lives. We fear the question, "Who does she think she is to desire like that?" from other women—and from ourselves.

And sometimes these questions do happen. Once, when I was sharing with a group of women what I longed for more of in my marriage, they all looked at me like I was insane. Several of them even said, "Are you kidding me? You have it all. Your life is perfect." After all, they said, they would give anything to have a marriage like mine. But their desires shouldn't influence mine. Desire is relative to one's life.

As I talked with these women, I initially had a flash of guilt for desiring more. But later that evening, after processing the experience with a friend, I realized I can't take directions for my life from women who do not have what I want. This was a catalyst moment for me and one that changed the game almost immediately. I started to shift who I spent time with and welcomed new, aligned friends into my life. I have since decided that I only have space for visionaries, big dreamers, people who walk with endless gratitude, and individuals who desire for more. Now you will only find me in the company of others where we are all so excited to share about our next steps, expansions, and what we are changing to create space for more abundance in our lives.

I am a woman who dreams big, hungers for more, and is ravenous for this life. This doesn't come from a place of greed but rather from awe and wonder for this life, this world, and the possibilities available to me. Almost every single year, without fail, I have some epic, wonderous thing I want to adventure into. And every year, while sharing with my husband, he stares back at me, silently, as if to say, "Here she goes again." At times, he has expressed frustration and exasperation at my huge desires. And each time,

I remind him that there is no chance of this ever changing for me. He has now accepted that my ravenous appetite for life is the essence of who I am. Many other people were continually perplexed and did not as easily accept my way of living. Most of them are no longer in my life.

It's critical to pay attention to anyone or anything that shames or vilifies you for wanting more from your life, relationships, career, and passions. Do not allow *their* narrative, fear, and limitations to define *your* life, because that self-betrayal is the worst of them all. You know who you are—act accordingly and fiercely protect your dreams.

The world perpetuates toxic positivity with sayings like "Live, Love, Laugh" and shames anything women want outside of traditional gender roles and minimal expectations for their life. After all, your desires can feel inconvenient, ridiculous, impossible, or embarrassing to the people in your life, including your parents, partner, and children. Even female friends, who have shut themselves off from desire, will try to hold you back or tell you your desires are unrealistic. They're wrong.

Desire is what makes life magical. But desire can feel illogical.

For many years, I made myself wrong for desiring so much. I now understand and honor that I am made this way, and with this knowing, have not allowed myself to be brainwashed into the gratitude trap. I am now as devoted to my desire practice as I am to my gratitude. It is the heartbeat of me. It's my essence. It's what lights me up from the inside out and keeps me feeling vibrant and exhilarated.

You can have that too. It starts with feeling into your desires.

FEELING INTO YOUR DESIRES

So let me ask you: What do you desire right now? this month? this year? next year?

Desire and pleasure are life force energy. Without them, we are simply going through the motions and not actually living into the magnificence of life. A life devoid of desire and pleasure is noticeable, like the lights are turned off. The essence of a woman comes alive when she is living into her desires and filling her daily life with pleasure. But so often, women stop dreaming, as if this were an art form reserved only for youth. The truth is, we forever get to recreate our lives and womanifest anything we desire.

We explored one way to begin to uncover your desires, through accessing your childhood memories. Now let's explore how to anchor into your body, access your internal GPS, and feel into your desires. When you close your eyes, circle your hips, and really feel into your body, what do you deeply desire? Circle the ones that apply.

- Days at the beach
- Walks in the woods
- More bubble baths
- More dancing
- More orgasms
- More delicious food
- More chocolate
- More eye contact
- More laughter
- More authenticity
- More bravery
- More success
- More money
- Soul purpose
- A luxury car
- A new home
- A new lover
- A cashmere wrap
- More hand-holding
- More candles
- More sensuality
- More embodiment
- Beautiful, raw sisterhood

Now, let me ask you a few questions to further uncover your desires. Answer these honestly. You may find it helpful to journal your reflections to create even deeper awareness.

- Does it feel easy to identify what you desire?
- Does it feel scary to long for more?

- Who in your life would find your desires inconvenient?
- Do you believe it benefits you to ignore your desires?
- What do you fear you will lose if you follow through on what you desire?
- How do you see your joy multiplying when you are living in your desire?
- If you were dying tomorrow, would you regret never fulfilling your desires?
- Do you feel worthy of these desires?
- Do you feel greedy for wanting your desires?
- Do you feel intimidated by the bigness of your desires?
- Do you find yourself asking, "What's even the point?"
- Do your desires feel impossible to cultivate in your current life?
- What stands in the way of each of the desires you circled?
- Is that really in the way or are you making excuses?

As you explore these questions, another big question will arise: What is the one *huge* desire you carry deep in your heart that you have had with you forever, but think it's ridiculous?

Quiet yourself. Be still. You know the answer. What is it?

As you embrace your desire, remember this: The only thing that's ridiculous about your desire is that you have been carrying it in silence. That desire was placed in your soul for you. It's part of your purpose.

With the knowledge of your desires, the next step is to begin to live into what your soul craves. Doing so can feel unsafe or too disruptive to your life. Stepping into your desires can cause you to let go of identities, people, and things in order to be in alignment with who you really are. Sometimes your soul's desire makes no sense, and it's something your mind resists. Here's where the illogical magic comes in, and you have to lean into self-trust. Your true soul desire is an energy that moves through you. It wants something for you. You might not know what that is initially. But you must surrender anyway.

Your desires are meant to be lived through you in your lifetime. Investing in yourself and your desires requires discipline, for which you will be rewarded exponentially.

This is where embodiment is important, as everything you desire starts within your body. When you're disconnected from your body or numb to your emotions, you can't possibly access your desires. But the truest version of you lives within your desires. You must get in touch with yourself often to access your deep desires—through dancing, journaling, being alone in nature, hip circles, pleasure, and other embodiment activities.

True desire feels unlike anything else in the universe. Even thinking about what you crave leaves you feeling an internal excitement, an aliveness that we are rarely able to access in our daily lives. Your desire is where your power lives! Plugging into your desires can light up your entire life. Desire is an undeniable call in your being, but to hear it you need to be fully honest with yourself. Desire is not concerned with the "how" but rather requires a trust in something greater than your own mind. You must put down your stories and fears and say yes to your desires again and again.

So tell me: What do you desire in your purpose? in your relationships? in sex? in community?

Pay attention to how alive you become when you talk about what you desire. Maybe you feel the swirl of butterflies in your stomach. The thrill of the idea. The buzz of something magnificent happening. The dizziness of excitement. Make sure to pay close attention to, and acknowledge, these feelings, as they are usually a sign that you have tapped into the essence of what you really want in your life. In the same way you would hear and validate a child who has a dream, you must do the same for yourself.

Along with self-validation, share with trusted loved ones and mentors what you are desiring to create or call in for your life. The people who deeply love and support you will want to see you move in the direction of your desires. The ones who don't will self-select out of your life or reveal the limitations of your relationship. Oftentimes, sharing our desires with others helps to expand the excitement and creates even more ideas about how to get started. Having accountability helps us to not quit on ourselves—another great reason to share your desires. Plus, desire often serves to inspire others to dream bigger for their lives as well.

When I work with groups of women and have them start to identify what they desire, something incredible happens. As one woman begins to share, her desire seems to have a thrilling effect on the others in the group. Almost immediately, each woman is eager to share what she wants for her life. It's incredible what is possible when surrounded by this kind of supportive energy, and that's why it is absolutely crucial to be in proximity to people who will not try to shut you down, minimize your feelings, or call your desires unrealistic and a waste of time.

I had a client who, after listening to the other women in my mastermind (an intensive group meeting that meets weekly for six months or so), became so inspired by all the ways in which they were creating change in their lives that she decided to borrow some of that energy and create change for her life as well. She was already an incredibly successful real estate agent who had been a leader in her industry for decades. She assumed that was what she would do forever, until she let herself tap into her deep desire.

When she really allowed herself to access her truth, she connected with a part of herself that loved flowers. She loved buying them, arranging them, and delivering them to friends. As we explored this further, she started to dream about turning her passion into a business. She allowed her excitement to fuel research into how she would build the business. She explored the legal requirements, spoke to others in the industry, and volunteered at local florist shops. Every time she started to feel like her idea was ridiculous, she would touch base with her heart. And every time, she felt an overwhelming confirmation that this was the direction for her.

She was fueled by desire! Every step kept leading to the next. Every time she would doubt the how, I encouraged her to keep moving in the direction of her desire, that each step would inform the next. The point wasn't the outcome—the point was for her to keep dreaming and know she can pivot at any time in her life. Every step gathers more data about future steps. I see so many people miss out on their desires because they say, "But how?" Desire does not care about how. It requires passion, trust, and action. When I last spoke with her, she was still working on these steps.

I've experienced the limitations of "how" in my own life. Just three years ago, my desire was to reach women around the world with my message. This seemed almost impossible. At the time, I was a psychologist leading local workshops. I didn't have any sort of major platform or any sign that my dream was possible.

But this desire had been building in me for years. It made my heart flutter with excitement.

The problem was that I would only allow myself to feel into it for a short while. When I did let myself dream, I would quickly bring my rational brain into the process, and within minutes, I'd convince myself that it was not only silly, but that I had missed my opportunity entirely, as I was close to fifty at the time. I also got stuck in the contentment loop and tried to convince myself that serving local women in my town was enough. Yet no matter how much I tried to rationalize this craving away, it always came back.

Desire has a way of wanting you to pay attention to it. There came a point where my desire to reach women globally was all I could think about, and I finally decided to go all in on my inexplicable desires. I had absolutely no idea how I was going to make it happen, but I knew I was committed to honoring and trusting that this desire was placed in me because it was made for me.

With this awareness, I decided to invest in myself and my vision every single day, and put zero focus on anything that pulled me away from my big, audacious plans to make a global impact with my work. Every time a doubt crept into my mind, I simply acknowledged that it was nothing more than my old limiting beliefs, and that I was no longer available to align with them.

I gave these limiting beliefs zero attention. This work allowed them to leave as fast as they came.

As I shifted my work toward my desire, I constantly asked myself: Is this thing you are doing, choosing, or deciding on taking you closer to, or further away, from your desires? Anything that took me further away needed to be released or readjusted. Some of the people around me changed as well.

I've said this once, but it bears repeating: It's necessary to pay attention to the company you keep when building the life of your dreams. Energy is contagious, and I had to make sure mine was protected and filled only with those who were of like mind in their own lives.

That's the other thing about desire: It will ask you to burn down and leave behind old beliefs, limited ways of being, and allegiances that keep you small. If you truly surrender to desire, it has the ability to remake you! But this path is not for the faint of heart. Maybe you don't desire to become internationally known, but you do want to create more emotional intimacy in your partnership. This will require you to become highly vulnerable—to lead with your heart wide open, to release old patterns of functioning with your partner, to try again every day, even when it feels terrifying. Desire is there to make our lives more beautiful.

To fulfill desire, you will have to become an energetic match for that desire. For example, I could never call in international reach with my work if I was terrified of being visible or afraid of criticism. Pay attention to whether what you desire and your beliefs may be a mismatch. Often, our old patterns get in the way of reaching what we crave.

If that's the case, begin with changing your beliefs and by teaching your nervous system to hold the frequency of what you want more of. This is the work you've been doing throughout this book—rewriting your internal script to step into the life you desire and deserve. Begin in your mind. And when you feel ready, you can experiment with welcoming in 1 percent of what you desire, slowly starting to make these desires feel safe in your mind and body.

Do not ignore the call. You were made for more. Give yourself full permission and approval to curate a life beyond your wildest dreams! Allow yourself to believe it is safe to have more, to receive what you so deeply desire. From here, you can curate the life of your desirous dreams.

Chapter 10

CURATE YOUR LIFE TO BECOME THE WOMAN OF YOUR DREAMS

"Freeing yourself was one thing, claiming
ownership of that freed self was another."

—TONI MORRISON, *BELOVED*

I WANT TO take a moment to celebrate you for making it through this book. I know, at times, the stories and concepts may have felt confronting and even outright triggering. Yet you continued on. You kept reading. You kept journeying. And I'd guess you kept at it because you see the opportunity for a more beautiful and truer female experience. A revolutionary womanhood.

When I teach to groups of women, I feel honored by the nods I see rippling across the room, whether it's a gathering of twelve or twelve hundred. Like you, they feel remembrance of the truth on a primal level. A truth that, in a patriarchal world, feels almost impossible to live into. And many women will choose not to even try. Sometimes staying unconscious is an easier path.

Those of us who choose to cross the bridge to deeper understanding, to all the magnificence that is available to us in this lifetime, can't simply turn around and go back. Doing so would feel like death. And so, we carry on.

That's been my experience—one of awareness, change, and carrying on. As we close our time together in this book, and you enter the next step of your journey, I want to share something personal. I've told many stories in this book, but I've waited until now to illustrate a profoundly private journey, and how I have navigated my own internalized patriarchy. I knew sharing this story and my own transformation required first guiding you through a full understanding of the concepts we've learned together. I will now take you through the entire arc of the book using my story to showcase what living this philosophy looks like in a real human life.

I'll start here: As I write this final chapter, I am one week post-op from breast explant surgery—at the end of a path I have been walking for entirely too long. Since the work of this book is a forever journey, a lifestyle, a new way of being a woman, we get to return to the concepts over and over again as we become braver. As we shed our conditioning and choose truth. Here is my story.

EXPLANTING PATRIARCHY

I was twenty-three years old, newly married, and in grad school in Los Angeles. While I had checked all the boxes I'd been taught to check—marriage, education—I still felt deeply self-conscious. The reason: my thin, zero-curve body. Then I met a few women in my grad program who had breast implants, and my curiosity was piqued. One afternoon, they openly shared about how much they loved their breasts, how sexy they felt, how all their clothes fit them so much better, and how their partners had never been happier with their bodies.

As I listened, I felt a flutter of excitement. Could I do something like that? I'd never even had any real awareness of the procedure, and certainly hadn't considered it for myself, until that one fated day. Looking back, I can now see how highly impressionable I was, because I stored this conversation as a "maybe someday" for myself.

That weekend, while I was putting pictures from our honeymoon into a photo album, I was caught off guard when I noticed myself in my swimsuit. Although I had seen these pictures before, this time I saw them through a more critical lens. As I held a photo of me, smiling, my new husband's arm around my waist, I couldn't take my eyes off my protruding chest bones and the almost concave shape of my chest. I felt embarrassed. I felt "less than" as a woman. Later that weekend, while at the beach with my husband, I fixated on all the women with larger breasts. They looked supple and sexy; by comparison, my body looked bony and harsh. As I studied their curves, I began to tell myself a story: that they had more beautiful and feminine bodies than I did.

Months passed, and I grew convinced that having larger breasts would make me happier in my body. I believed I would feel more confident, both naked and clothed, and look more feminine and sexier. One evening, while sitting at our dining table finishing dinner, I announced my desire to my husband. I listed my reasons behind the choice. He was confused as to why and asked a few questions to see if I had really thought this decision through, and very soon he, too, supported my decision. And just like that, I started looking for a plastic surgeon, booked my augmentation, and even as they rolled me back for surgery, acted as if it were a benign decision.

After the surgery, I was thrilled. I loved my new breasts and felt I had made a choice from a place of power. Now, I wish I could go back and wrap my arms around that young woman who let her body be cut into, who allowed foreign objects to be inserted into it, who risked her health and life for bigger breasts and what she thought was a sexier profile. Who believed the lie that being sexy had anything to do with one's shape to begin with, who chose to inflict pain on herself rather than unearth the pain from within.

I lived in my false empowerment for a few years, until I learned I was unexpectedly pregnant. That news changed my feelings about having implants and I was immediately flooded with regret. What if I could not breastfeed?

To assuage my guilt and figure out how to feed my baby, I started researching and gathered every single piece of information I could find. I even joined an online group of women who had been successful with nursing their babies after augmentation. Still, I felt overwhelming feelings of guilt and shame for my choice. At times, the regret was all-consuming.

I wish I could go back and wrap my arms around that young woman who let her body be cut into, who allowed foreign objects to be inserted into her it, who risked her health and life for bigger breasts and what she thought was a sexier profile.

At this point, my life took a drastic turn. I had my doctorate in psychology, was in private practice, and was deeply educated on human behavior. My professional exposure and diverse training had taught me so much—and yet I had no idea about the world I was about to step into and how it would forever change the trajectory of my life and beliefs.

At four months pregnant, I joined a local La Leche League, a group for breastfeeding women. During lunch breaks from work, I would attend the meetings: listening, learning, and asking questions. I'd never known a woman who breastfed, and I knew I needed to do more than simply read about breastfeeding or chat in online forums. More than anything, I needed proximity to women who were nursing and a support system once my baby was born.

In these meetings, I also learned about natural childbirth, midwives, and classes that my husband and I could attend. I signed us up for a twelve-week intensive class, during which my eyes were opened to the profound power of women and our bodies. That course is also where my fury was born, as I grew angry that the beauty of birth was not the mainstream story. Most stories were riddled with fear and had no real connection to the power of birthing and the female body. I started to see the influence of the storyteller, the patriarchy, and the medical systems that make millions as they profit from perpetuated terror.

Fast-forward two babies born and two years of breastfeeding later, and I began to search for a doctor who could perform an explant surgery. I wanted these foreign objects out of my body. I wanted to be free of the worry. I desired to no longer have my heart chakra blocked, and I craved my natural body. After three separate consultations, I grew disheartened after hearing "it's impossible," "the result will be devastating," and "you will be deformed." I was infuriated at myself for having ever gotten into this situation to begin with and felt trapped in this horrible decision I had made.

I finally resorted to having them removed and replaced with the absolute smallest implants on the market. Due to the extensive breastfeeding, my skin had stretched badly and I needed a breast lift in order to replace the implants. I tried to make peace with this decision and move on with my life, but I must admit I was haunted by the choice.

As the years passed, the cognitive dissonance grew to the point I could no longer feel peaceful about my decision. The only true resolve would be to have the implants completely out of my body. They felt like foreign invaders, and I was on a mission to find a doctor who could hear me and help me. Not only did I find a doctor, but I found one whose entire practice is explant surgery. The majority of his patients have breast implant illness and must explant because they are so sick. Many of the women were suffering from fatigue, memory and concentration problems, joint pain, gastrointestinal issues, and other debilitating symptoms. I was fortunate to not be sick from my implants, but the lack of urgency also meant I had to join the almost two-year waiting list so those who were sick could take the priority spots.

Finally, my explant day arrived. As I waited, I witnessed female rebirth. Each time I watched a woman being wheeled out into the recovery room after their surgery, I felt another victory for all women, as if the female collective was getting a bit freer from all the conditioning, pressure, and lies. And as I was wheeled back for my own surgery, I felt a reclamation so powerful, I wept until the anesthesia took hold. On the drive home, and all through the night, I continued to sob. My husband initially assumed I was crying in pain, but I shared with him that my tears were a mixture of grief for the young version of me who made that decision, for the journey in between, and for the woman I had fully stepped into.

Here I sit, one week after surgery. And for the first time in twenty-seven years, I feel the most aligned, free, and at home in my body. Let us now explore, using the material from this book, how I traveled this path.

A FRAMEWORK FOR ROOTING INTO ONESELF

I've talked about how, as a young woman, I fell into the trap of feeling less worthy, less feminine, and less desirable because I created a story that a flat chest was not appealing. I believed surgery would provide me with more femininity, more beauty, more feeling like an actual woman.

Before my implant surgery, I had no connection to any feminine practices. Like most women, I was raised in a patriarchal family, had a patriarchal career, and had no role models for sourcing from within. And I certainly knew absolutely nothing about embodiment. While I made the choice to get implants from a disempowered place, I had convinced myself it was from a place of self-agency and internal power. A few years later, when I became pregnant, I was exposed to more embodied ways of living and the art of ancient feminine practices. From there, my whole world expanded.

Let's look at each of the steps I took to get to where I am today, each of which you've already been exposed to throughout this book. I'll summarize my journey so you can use my experience to guide your own.

Take radical responsibility.

With my new lens and eyes wide open, I became a radically responsible woman who began questioning everything I once believed. I questioned rules, structures, and systems. I bucked almost all of what I uncovered as I became more educated. Ultimately, I began to listen to and trust my intuition.

Become a self-led woman.

I started to lead myself in almost every single aspect of my life, and I stopped looking to other people and systems to give me directions to my own existence. I simultaneously outgrew the need to explain my life choices. This is where the great shift happened and I became the curator of my life. I was no longer unconscious to the machine of toxic beauty culture and patriarchy. I would no longer be a helpless princess. I became committed to building a life that felt deeply aligned with my internal knowing, regardless of what others were choosing.

Tune out the world's messaging and turn on your inner wisdom.

My family, friends, colleagues, and medical doctors all began to think I was "too much" and that I took everything too seriously. This is when I doubled down on my beliefs and became immune to the world's messaging and advice, including from family, friends, and other people who didn't have the kind of life I aspired to have. I stopped putting blind faith into so-called leaders. I shifted my focus toward listening to, and trusting, my own voice. I became my own authority.

Clean up and detox what you absorb.

In order to quiet the outside opinions and rely on my inner wisdom, I had to make fundamental changes in my life. This included becoming mindful of what I watched, what I listened to, and which accounts I followed on social media. I started reading books that felt aligned with my soul and didn't worry what others might think if they saw those books on my coffee table. I listened to music that spoke to my heart. I started drinking less alcohol, started eating more whole organic foods, and signed up for activities I felt drawn to, even if nobody else I knew was participating. I started to deeply study and investigate systems at large in an effort to fully understand why being a woman never felt safe and sacred—and to learn how to make it so.

Decide who you want to be.

I decided I wanted to be a woman who made deeply informed decisions. I decided I wanted to be a woman who didn't conform or swallow her truth— one who said the hard thing every single time. I decided I was not meant to be an object to the patriarchy, or to be pleasing to make others feel comfortable. I decided the way I looked, thought, and felt was more important than anyone's opinion about me. I decided I wanted to stop betraying myself and my truth. And then I lived in alignment with that decision.

Begin living now as the woman you want to become.

Once I decided who I wanted to become, I started adjusting every aspect of my life. I reviewed my beliefs, behaviors, and relationships. I asked myself: Does this align with who I want to be? Will this support my efforts to get to the life I desire to create? Where can I make adjustments? What needs to change? Who do I need to release? What and who will hinder me on my journey?

I answered each of these questions honestly. And with awareness of the woman I wanted to become, I made the changes needed to become her.

Build a life of self-trust and self-approval.

I decided I would trust and honor my inner wisdom, even when everyone around me was making completely different choices. I stopped listening to the opinions of others, especially those who didn't have the life I wanted to create. I learned how to feel for the truth inside of myself rather than be influenced by outside sources. And I built even more trust in myself every time I showed up for my needs—when I didn't abandon my truth and when I spoke from my heart. I became free once I decided the only approval I ever needed was my own.

Remember you are worthy.

With the endless messaging coming every day at women, threatening a sense of worthiness, it's an act of resistance to not give these messages any power. I did three things to assure I stayed anchored in my Queen energy, including feelings of self-worth: First, I followed only those social accounts that were uplifting and inspiring. Second, I surrounded myself only with women of a similar mindset and I paid attention to how I felt after every interaction. If I felt uninspired or exhausted after being with someone, I trusted that my body was showing me signs that we were not an energetic match, and I would adjust accordingly. And third, I became bulletproof in what I allowed to be absorbed into my consciousness as absolute truths. I recognized that almost all marketing targeted to women is fear-based, meant to keep us enslaved to toxic beauty culture. I refused to see media and marketing messaging as anything more than that. In essence, I became immune to the bullshit.

Become the leading lady of your life.

As women, we are conditioned to put everyone before ourselves and to be selfless in all our actions. We often feel guilty about prioritizing ourselves. I noticed that so much of my life and energy was spent giving to others that there was rarely any time left for myself. I recognized that basing my existence on only being a supporting character in everyone else's lives was not going to lead to fulfillment. Eventually, I realized, I would feel resentful. I also didn't want my loved ones to feel the burden of my unlived life. I've seen countless parents do this to their children; I didn't want my kids to carry that weight.

From this awareness emerged a life-changing truth: I had to be the one to prioritize myself! So with my list of desires, I started to live as the main character of my life, which meant no more waiting for the perfect time or putting off self-prioritization until after everyone else's needs were met. From this energy, I felt liberated, excited for each day, and balanced in a way I had never experienced.

Lead your life with intention and make beautiful meaning.

I knew I didn't have to accept what society or the world assigns as meaning to things in life, including beauty, success, aging, and pleasure. Through the lens of radical responsibility, I decided to be the meaning-maker for my own life. As I tried on this way of being, I was astounded with how free I felt to make new choices. It was fun to be in this energy! As I continued to live with intention and make beautiful meaning, I expanded what I saw as possible for all aspects of my life, career, and relationships.

Live the story you want to tell at the end of your life.

Rather than living in fear, doubt, and scarcity, I decided to live my life rooted in being bold, confident, and abundant. To do this, I considered all the things I would regret if I found out I was dying tomorrow. Living this way has made my life feel more urgent and allowed me to get into inspired action. Now, rather than focus on all that could go wrong, I put my energy into all that will go right.

Through each of these points of awareness, action steps, and areas of growth, you get to become the woman of your dreams. You get to decide how you want to show up. And as you change your own life, you get to become your own muse, to light an inner fire that will burn brightly for others. Because while one woman changing is powerful, many women changing is a movement. As you grow that inner flame, as you step more fully into your dream life, as you become your own muse, you may feel the calling to reach out to the women around you and lift them up too. To share your story. Who knows—maybe I'll be reading your book someday!

The honor of my life is helping you step more fully into yours. Not creating something new for you but helping you unearth who you already are, step fully into her, and live as a freed woman. This work is about loving yourself. Knowing your own body. Trusting your inner wisdom. Navigating the world with a knowing no one can take from you.

So let me ask you: What story do you want to create? What do you want to make your one and only precious life mean? Starting now, you can continue this journey and create a life that is divinely yours.

WOMANIFESTO

I believe my feminine is divinely powerful.

I believe self-love is my greatest love.

I believe and trust my body.

I believe my own opinion is most important for my life.

I believe soul care is the greatest way to nourish myself.

I believe aging is a spiritual journey.

I believe my body holds infinite wisdom.

I trust my greatest guidance comes from my deep intuition.

I trust the cycles of my feminine body and merge with them.

I trust my desires are mine to fully claim.

I trust my self-leadership.

I trust that my truth sets me free.

I trust the worthiness of my voice.

I trust that abundance in all its glorious forms is available to me.

I am a woman who finds pleasure in all things.

I am a woman who sources from within.

I am a woman who self-approves.

I am a woman who does not shrink to make others feel comfortable.

I am a woman who waits for no one.

I am a woman who celebrates.

I am a woman who craves and claims more.

I know that my expansion heals my lineage.

I know that my body is a temple.

I know that my sensuality is my superpower.

I know that I can transmute my pain into my passion.

I know that I was born worthy.

I know that I am a miracle.

I know it is my responsibility to curate the life I dream of.

TEN QUESTIONS FOR BOOK CLUB

1. What did your mother, or another female role model, teach you about what it means to be a woman? Has that definition of womanhood become an obstacle or support on your path?

2. What is your relationship with aging? Does your current belief system around aging serve you?

3. Where did you feel triggered in the book? Where did you feel seen?

4. What harmful beliefs about your body do you hold? What would releasing these lies look like for you?

5. How has toxic beauty culture influenced your life, and what lies have you previously fallen for that were exposed in this book? What would releasing these lies look like for you?

6. What change would you like to see for the next generations of women—your daughter or any other younger women you love?

7. If you were to step into revolutionary womanhood, which relationships—family, friends, colleagues, acquaintances—might be impacted, and how?

8. Do all of your female friendships feel safe and supportive? Do you feel uplifted by every friend? If not, what beliefs or behaviors do you want to change within your friendships?

9. How can you trust your body more? What are some immediate rituals you can integrate in order to connect with your body?

10. If you knew you wouldn't lose anyone or be criticized, and that you'd be completely safe expressing yourself, what desires would you boldly claim for your life?

NOTES

Chapter 1

1. Sumathi Reddy, "For Women, Midlife Brain Fog Is Real. Here's Why," *Wall Street Journal,* March 20, 2023, https://www.wsj.com/articles/ brain-fog-perimenopause-midlife-women-memory-problems-forgetting-menopause-77e5cb95.

2. Sharom Romm, "Beauty Through History: The Changing Ideal," *Washington Post*, January 26, 1987, https://www.washingtonpost.com/ archive/lifestyle/wellness/1987/01/27/beauty-through-history/301f7256-0f6b-403e-abec-f36c0a3ec313/.

3. "Body and Beauty Standards," The Body Project, Bradley University, last updated March 26, 2021, https://www.bradley.edu/sites/ bodyproject/standards/#:~:text=According%20to%20Hoff%20 (2019)%2C,without%20using%20extremely%20unhealthy%20means.

4. "Body Measurements," National Center for Health Statistics, Centers for Disease Control and Prevention, last reviewed September 10, 2021, https://www.cdc.gov/nchs/fastats/body-measurements.htm.

5. Erica Åberg, Iida Kukkonen, and Outi Sarpila, "From Double to Triple Standards of Ageing. Perceptions of Physical Appearance at the Intersections of Age, Gender and Class," *Journal of Aging Studies* 55 (December 2020): https://www.sciencedirect.com/science/article/pii/ S0890406520300463.

6. Achim Berg et al., "The Beauty Market in 2023: A Special State of Fashion Report," McKinsey & Company, May 22, 2023, https://www.mckinsey.com/industries/retail/our-insights/the-beauty-market-in-2023-a-special-state-of-fashion-report.

7. Marta Kowal et al., "Predictors of Enhancing Human Physical Attractiveness: Data from 93 Countries," *Evolution and Human Behavior* 43, no. 6 (November 2022): 455–474, https://www.sciencedirect.com/science/article/pii/S1090513822000472.

Chapter 2

1. Susan C. Lawrence and Kae Bendixen, "His and Hers: Male and Female Anatomy in Anatomy Texts for U.S. Medical Students, 1890–1989," *Social Science and Medicine* 35, no. 7 (October 1992): 925–934, https://www.sciencedirect.com/science/article/abs/pii/0277953692901072.

2. Melissa Fyfe, "Get Cliterate: How a Melbourne Doctor Is Redefining Female Sexuality," *Sydney Morning Herald*, December 8, 2018, https://www.smh.com.au/lifestyle/health-and-wellness/get-cliterate-how-a-melbourne-doctor-is-redefining-female-sexuality-20181203-p50jvv.html.

3. Helen E. O'Connell, Kalavampara V. Sanjeevan, and John M. Hutson, "Anatomy of the Clitoris," *The Journal of Urology* 174 (October 2005): 1189–1195, https://edisciplinas.usp.br/pluginfile.php/7538561/mod_resource/content/1/O%E2%80%99Connell%20et%20al.%20%282005%29%20-%20%20Anatomia%20do%20clit%C3%B3ris.pdf.

4. Fyfe, "Get Cliterate."

5. Google Scholar, list of articles referencing "clitoris orgasm," accessed April 14, 2024, https://scholar.google.com/scholar?q=clitoris+orgasm&hl=en&as_sdt=0%2C5&as_ylo=2022&as_yhi=2024.

6. Laurie Mintz, "The Orgasm Gap: Simple Truth & Sexual Solutions," *Psychology Today*, October 4, 2015, https://www.psychologytoday.com/us/blog/stress-and-sex/201510/the-orgasm-gap-simple-truth-sexual-solutions.

7. Rainey Horwitz, "Vaginal Speculum (after 1800)," *Embryo Project Encyclopedia*, Arizona State University, last modified September 11, 2023, https://embryo.asu.edu/pages/vaginal-speculum-after-1800#:~:text=Sims%20used%20a%20bent%20spoon,in%20the%20twenty%2Dfirst%20century.

8. Camila Domonoske, "'Father of Gynecology,' Who Experimented on Slaves, No Longer on Pedestal in NYC," *The Two-Way,* NPR, April 17, 2018, https://www.npr.org/sections/thetwo-way/2018/04/17/603163394/-father-of-gynecology-who-experimented-on-slaves-no-longer-on-pedestal-in-nyc.

9. J. Marion Sims, *The Story of My Life* (New York: D. Appleton and Company, 1884), 231.

10. Domonoske, "'Father of Gynecology.'"

11. Claire Breen, "Women behind Speculum Redesign Say We Need Gynecological Tools Designed by People with Vaginas," *The Washington Post*, October 12, 2017, https://www.washingtonpost.com/gender-identity/women-behind-speculum-redesign-say-we-need-gynecological-tools-designed-by-people-with-vaginas/.

12. Horwitz, "Vaginal Speculum."

13. Joanna Thompson, "No One Studied Menstrual Product Absorbency Realistically until Now," *Scientific American*, August 22, 2023, https://www.scientificamerican.com/article/no-one-studied-menstrual-product-absorbency-realistically-until-now/.

14. Aristotle, *Politics*, Perseus Digital Library, Tufts University, 1252a, https://www.perseus.tufts.edu/hopper/text?doc=Perseus:text:1999.01.0058:book=1.

15. Aristotle, *Generation of Animals*, Digital Loeb Classical Library, 174–175, https://www.loebclassics.com/view/aristotle-generation_animals/1942/pb_LCL366.175.xml.

16. *Oxford Languages*, s.v. "history," Google, accessed May 21, 2024, https://www.google.com/search?sca_esv=565026230&sxsrf=AM9HkKkJ8WBPiTrtlOwRM5rPWpXJaic65g:1694681554384&q=history&si=ALGXSlZCBshTM3a3nPTSW0d1OmQerpr770VzC0Fn1MxJQGxUMXPF3LRHy8-66AkYZLSocRhdQJe61poNMnkXUq6P-aPXSqPiXA%3D%3D&expnd=1&sa=X&ved=2ahUKEwi-urng3KmBAxUnkokEHa9ZAnsQ2v4IegQIGBBq&biw=1377&bih=728&dpr=1.

17. Stacy L. Smith, Katherine Pieper, and Sam Wheeler, *Inclusion in the Director's Chair: Analysis of Director Gender and Race/Ethnicity Across the 1,600 Top Films from 2007 to 2022*, USC Annenberg Inclusion Initiative, January 2023, https://deadline.com/wp-content/uploads/2023/01/Inclusion-In-The-Director-Chair-2022-USC-Study.pdf; "Violence in

the Media and Entertainment (Position Paper)," All Policies, American Academy of Family Physicians (AAFP), accessed May 2, 2024, https://www.aafp.org/about/policies/all/violence-media-entertainment.html.

18. PR Newswire, "The Highest Grossing Film of 2023 Worldwide BARBIE," Warner Bros. Home Entertainment, September 5, 2023, https://www.prnewswire.com/news-releases/the-highest-grossing-film-of-2023-worldwide-barbie-301917178.html#:~:text=Gerwig%20 directed%20%22Barbie%22%20from%20a,based%20on%20Barbie%20 by%20Mattel.&text=%22Barbie%22%20has%20taken%20the%20 box,grossing%20film%20in%20Warner%20Bros.

19. Caroline Criado Perez, *Invisible Women: Exposing Data Bias in a World Designed for Men* (New York: Abrams Press, 2019).

20. Jeannie Kopstein and Mariah Espada, "The Staggering Economic Impact of Taylor Swift's Eras Tour," *Time*, August 23 2023, https://time.com/6307420/taylor-swift-eras-tour-money-economy/; Abha Bhattarai, Rachel Lerman, and Emily Sabens, "The Economy (Taylor's Version)," *The Washington Post*, October 13, 2023, https://www.washingtonpost.com/business/2023/10/13/taylor-swift-eras-tour-money-jobs/.

21. Ana Faguy, "Beyoncé's Renaissance Tour Brings in Half-Billion Dollars—But These Singers Made Even More," Business, *Forbes*, October 3, 2023, accessed January 3, 2024, https://www.forbes.com/sites/anafaguy/2023/10/03/beyoncs-renaissance-tour-brings-in-half-billion-dollars-but-these-singers-made-even-more/?sh=711f675a4e72.

22. Rayka Zehtabchi and Shaandiin Tome, "When a Girl's First Period Calls for Celebration, Not Stigma," *New York Times*, November 1, 2022, https://www.nytimes.com/2022/11/01/opinion/karuk-indigenous-celebration-menstruation-ceremony.html.

23. Mary Annette Pember, "'Honoring Our Monthly Moons': Some Menstruation Rituals Give Indigenous Women Hope," Rewire News Group, February 20, 2019, https://rewirenewsgroup.com/2019/02/20/monthly-moons-menstruation-rituals-indigenous-women/.

24. Audre Lorde, "The Master's Tools Will Never Dismantle the Master's House," in *Sister Outsider* (Berkeley, CA: The Crossing Press, 1984; reprint 2007).

Chapter 4

1. Naomi Fry, "And Just Like That . . .Carrie's Back! Sarah Jessica Parker Opens Up About a Grand Return," *Vogue*, November 7, 2021, https://www.vogue.com/article/sarah-jessica-parker-cover-december-2021.

2. Katie Couric, host, *Next Question with Katie Couric* (podcast), "Lisa LaFlamme's Silver Lining," March 30, 2023, https://www.youtube.com/watch?v=KhxJgUKAwo4&t=1s.

3. Homer Swei et al., "Survey Finds Use of Personal Care Products Up Since 2004—What That Means for Your Health," Environmental Working Group (EWG), July 26, 2023, https://www.ewg.org/research/survey-finds-use-personal-care-products-2004-what-means-your-health.

Chapter 5

1. cteintrocommercials, *Run Like a Girl*, YouTube, October 25, 2014, https://www.youtube.com/watch?v=qtDMyGjYlMg.

2. National Organization for Women, "Get the Facts," https://now.org/now-foundation/love-your-body/love-your-body-whats-it-all-about/get-the-facts/.

3. Mel Rising Dawn Cordeiro, "Body Image Issues Affect Many, Adolescent Girls and Adult Women Especially," Ocean State Stories, The Pell Center, Salve Regina University, June 27, 2023, https://oceanstatestories.org/body-image-issues-affect-many-adolescent-girls-and-adult-women-especially/#:~:text=According%20to%20the%20National%20Organization,time%20the%20girls%20reach%2017.

Chapter 6

1. Katharina Buchholz, "This Is How Female Representation Is Rising Across the Film Industry," World Economic Forum, March 31, 2022, https://www.weforum.org/agenda/2022/03/number-of-women-in-film-industry-rises-slowly.

2. Kate Kersey, Antonia C. Lyons, and Fiona Hutton, "Alcohol and Drinking within the Lives of Midlife Women: A Meta-Study Systematic Review," *International Journal of Drug Policy* 99 (January 2022), https://pubmed.ncbi.nlm.nih.gov/34653766/.

Chapter 7

1. Rachel Hoskins, "Life Cycle of a Tree: How Trees Grow," Woodland Trust, June 24, 2019, https://www.woodlandtrust.org.uk/blog/2019/06/tree-lifecycle/#:~:text=A%20tree%20becomes%20mature%20when,productivity%20around%2080%2D120%20years.

2. Mary Annette Pember, "'Honoring Our Monthly Moons': Some Menstruation Rituals Give Indigenous Women Hope," Rewire News Group, February 20, 2019, https://rewirenewsgroup.com/2019/02/20/monthly-moons-menstruation-rituals-indigenous-women/.

3. Sanjay Mishra, "The Menstrual Cycle Can Reshape Your Brain," *National Geographic*, February 7, 2024, https://www.nationalgeographic.com/premium/article/menstruation-brain-women-reshape.

4. "Method of Delivery," National Center for Health Statistics, Centers for Disease Control and Prevention, last reviewed April 9, 2024, https://www.cdc.gov/nchs/fastats/delivery.htm.

5. Munira Z. Gunja, Evan D. Gumas, and Reginald D. Williams II, *U.S. Health Care from a Global Perspective, 2022: Accelerating Spending, Worsening Outcomes* (brief), The Commonwealth Fund, January 31, 2023, https://www.commonwealthfund.org/publications/issue-briefs/2023/jan/us-health-care-global-perspective-2022.

6. *Online Etymology Dictionary,* s.v. "menopause *(n.),*" updated August 1, 2020, https://www.etymonline.com/word/menopause.

7. Cleveland Clinic, s.v. "menopause," last reviewed October 5, 2021, https://my.clevelandclinic.org/health/diseases/21841-menopause.

8. Cleveland Clinic, s.v. "perimenopause," last reviewed October 5, 2021, https://my.clevelandclinic.org/health/diseases/21608-perimenopause.

9. Cleveland Clinic, s.v. "menopause."

10. "What Is Menopause?," National Institute on Aging, National Institutes of Health, content reviewed September 30, 2021, https://www.nia.nih.gov/health/menopause/what-menopause#transition.

11. Andrea Petersen, "Why So Many Women in Middle Age Are on Antidepressants," *Wall Street Journal*, April 2, 2022, https://www.wsj.com/articles/why-so-many-middle-aged-women-are-on-antidepressants-11648906393.

12. Clarissa Brincat, "Why Is the Clit So Sensitive? Thanks to Over 10,000 Nerves, First Real Count Finds," Medical News Today, November 3, 2022, https://www.medicalnewstoday.com/articles/why-is-the-clit-so-sensitive-thanks-to-over-10000-nerves-first-real-count-finds.

Chapter 8

1. On yoga for men, see: Thomas Buch, "Yoga Was Invented by Men—for Men," *Maniphesto*, https://maniphesto.com/yoga-was-invented-by-men-for-men/#:~:text=For%20hundreds%20of%20years%20and,powerful%20challenge%20for%20one%20self.

2. Chelcey Adami, "Christopher Gardner on Netflix's *You Are What You Eat*," Stanford Report, January 18, 2024, https://news.stanford.edu/report/2024/01/18/qa-christopher-gardner-featured-netflixs-eat/.

Chapter 9

1. Summer Allen, *The Science of Gratitude* (white paper prepared for the John Templeton Foundation by the Greater Good Science Center at UC Berkeley, May 2018), https://ggsc.berkeley.edu/images/uploads/GGSC-JTF_White_Paper-Gratitude-FINAL.pdf?_ga=2.51257770.246418475.1638563377-157927757.1638563377.

ACKNOWLEDGMENTS

I WANT TO express my deepest appreciation to my family, who not only supported my endless hours dedicated to this book but has also engaged in many decades of thought-provoking and heart-opening conversations. Thank you for your constant willingness to sit for hours around the table and travel to the center of difficult topics without ever turning away. I am in awe of what we have created.

Stacy Ennis, you are a literary dream come true. Having your eyes, heart, and expertise on this book for the past year made the experience absolutely incredible. Thank you for teaching me how to take my philosophy from my heart to the pages.

Diana, you are the megaphone to my heart. From day one, you saw the bigness of my message and the urgency to get it into the hearts and homes of women around the world, and you have done exactly that. I am forever grateful for your passion and expertise.

To every single client, both past and present, who trusted me to be a part of their life journeys. Every one of your stories is a masterpiece. Thank you for your willingness to reach for more.

ABOUT THE AUTHOR

DR. AMANDA HANSON, known as The Midlife Muse, is a doctor of psychology, speaker, and author renowned for her transformative work in redefining womanhood. Her teachings have reached millions of women across the world—and have sparked a global movement of women living truer, more beautiful lives.

Throughout her twenty-five-year career as a psychologist, Dr. Amanda's work has exposed the patriarchal structures that keep women small, quiet, and at war with their bodies. Her approach combines clinical psychology with proven ancient holistic methods and sees the female body and mind as harmonious systems. Both must be in balance for wellness.

Alongside her work, Dr. Amanda is a mother of four, a wife, and an activist who strongly stands for inclusion, diversity, and equality. She chose the natural aging journey because she believes that aging is a spiritual experience when approached with a profound sense of self-worth.